Praise for
SUPPLEMENT YOUR PRESCRIPTION

For every dollar we spend on prescription drugs,
we spend a dollar to fix a complication. Understanding
how nutritional supplements affect these drugs
could make them safer and more effective.

—MEHMET OZ, M.D., PROFESSOR OF SURGERY AT COLUMBIA UNIVERSITY
AND BEST-SELLING AUTHOR OF *YOU: THE OWNER'S MANUAL* AND *YOU: ON A DIET*

As Dr. Cass makes crystal clear, what you don't know
can hurt you. In this age of pharmaceutical-based medicine,
this book is a must-read for patients and physicians alike.

—JULIAN WHITAKER, M.D., FOUNDER OF THE WHITAKER WELLNESS INSTITUTE
AND AUTHOR OF THE *HEALTH & HEALING* NEWSLETTER

Medications have been reported to kill over 200,000
Americans a year, with most physicians sadly being
clueless about how to avoid this. Dr. Cass once again
does an outstanding job teaching us how to reclaim our
birthright of optimal health—easily and naturally!

—JACOB TEITELBAUM, M.D., MEDICAL DIRECTOR OF THE FIBROMYALGIA AND
FATIGUE CENTERS AND AUTHOR OF *FROM FATIGUED TO FANTASTIC*!

This subject is so timely and the implications
so powerful, that Dr. Cass's new book deserves
to be read by everybody taking prescription meds,
and more importantly, by their doctors.

—ANN LOUISE GITTLEMAN, PH.D., C.N.S., AWARD-WINNING AUTHOR OF
THE FAT FLUSH PLAN AND *BEFORE THE CHANGE*

Supplement Your Prescription breaks new ground in the previously unexplored terrain of how nutrients are depleted by prescriptive drugs and how to use them together wisely. A boon for both conventional and integrative medicine, this book eliminates the confusion and the guesswork. Both physician and patient will benefit tremendously from Dr. Cass's research, insight, and practical application.

—GERALD M. LEMOLE, M.D., CHIEF OF CARDIOVASCULAR SURGERY AT CHRISTIANA CARE HEALTH SERVICES, AND AUTHOR OF *THE HEALING DIET*

From a recognized leader in the field of integrative medicine, *Supplement Your Prescription* is a vital resource to help patients avoid drug-nutrient depletion, and even enhance the benefits of their drugs with synergistic nutrients. A must-read!

—RONALD L. HOFFMAN, M.D., MEDICAL DIRECTOR OF THE HOFFMAN CENTER AND AUTHOR OF *HOW TO TALK WITH YOUR DOCTOR* (*ABOUT COMPLEMENTARY AND ALTERNATIVE MEDICINE*)

This book empowers people to take control of their health by knowing what their medications are really doing. It contains a huge amount of information, like an encyclopedia, but an easy read. A must read for everyone taking a medication!

—DWIGHT LUNDELL, M.D., HEART SURGEON AND AUTHOR OF *THE CURE FOR HEART DISEASE*

If you are taking prescription medications, you must protect yourself, and Dr. Cass tells you how to do it.

—STEPHEN SINATRA, M.D., MEDICAL DIRECTOR OF THE NEW ENGLAND HEART & LONGEVITY CENTER AND CO-AUTHOR OF *REVERSE HEART DISEASE NOW*

This book is a must-read for anyone who takes prescription drugs and doesn't want to suffer needless side effects.

—MARCUS LAUX, N.D., AUTHOR OF *NATURALLY WELL TODAY* NEWSLETTER

SUPPLEMENT
YOUR
PRESCRIPTION

What Your Doctor Doesn't
Know About Nutrition

Hyla Cass, M.D.

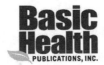

Basic Health
PUBLICATIONS, INC.

The information contained in this book is based upon the research and personal and professional experiences of the author. It is not intended as a substitute for consulting with your physician or other healthcare provider. Any attempt to diagnose and treat an illness should be done under the direction of a healthcare professional.

The publisher does not advocate the use of any particular healthcare protocol but believes the information in this book should be available to the public. The publisher and author are not responsible for any adverse effects or consequences resulting from the use of the suggestions, preparations, or procedures discussed in this book. Should the reader have any questions concerning the appropriateness of any procedures or preparation mentioned, the author and the publisher strongly suggest consulting a professional healthcare advisor.

Basic Health Publications, Inc.
28812 Top of the World Drive
Laguna Beach, CA 92651
949-715-7327 • www.basichealthpub.com

Library of Congress Cataloging-in-Publication Data
Cass, Hyla.
   Supplement your prescription : what your doctor doesn't know about nutrition / Hyla Cass.
     p. cm.
   Includes bibliographical references and index.
   ISBN 978-1-59120-227-1
  1. Drugs—Side effects—Popular works. 2. Dietary supplements—Popular works. 3. Nutrition—Popular works. 4. Alternative medicine—Popular works. I. Title.
   RM302.5.C38 2007
   615'.7042--dc22

                                                                    2007036820

Editor: Cheryl Hirsch
Typesetting/Interior design: Gary A. Rosenberg
Cover design: Mike Stromberg

Printed in the United States of America

10   9   8   7   6   5   4   3   2   1

Contents

Acknowledgments

Needless to say, extensive projects are rarely a one-person show, so there are many people I wish to thank for their help with this book. Not in any particular order, I am grateful to Norman Goldfind, my generous, kind, and very able publisher; Melissa Block, who skillfully, cheerfully, and reliably helped me write this book; and Cheryl Hirsch, my editor, who was there whenever I needed her, with creative suggestions and an admirable sense of organization.

Thanks to Jim LaValle and Deirdre Allen who generously shared their health information website (www.nhiondemand.com). Many other friends and colleagues answered questions, reviewed writing, and were available whenever I needed them. They include my old friend and prolific author, Stevanne Auerbach (a.k.a. Dr. Toy); Nan Fuchs (editor and writer, *Women's Health Letter*), who's been there unfailingly; my ongoing cheerleader, Siri Khalsa (publisher, *Nutrition News*); Marcia Zimmerman (author, *7-Color Cuisine*); and nutrition pioneer and writer par excellence, Betty Kamen, who valiantly stepped in when I needed her.

I deeply thank my parents for their ongoing love and support throughout my life: my late father, Isadore Cass, M.D., who taught me by example how to be a skilled and caring physician; and my mother, Miriam Cass, who loves my books, and still gets excited when she or her friends see me on TV or when I am quoted in the news. I thank my three sisters and brothers-in-law who give me constant moral support, and, most especially, my amazing daughter, Dr. Alison Schur, who, along with her adoring and adorable husband Seth, provide me with joy and great advice. I feel blessed to have such wonderful support in my life and to be able to communicate to others all I have learned, especially from my patients, who are my best teachers.

Introduction

We are taking prescription drugs in increasing numbers. Nearly 50 percent of American adults take at least one prescription medication, and nearly 20 percent take three or more. Over half of sixty-five-year olds take three prescription drugs or more daily. There has also been a steady and dramatic increase in money spent on prescriptions—nearly $200 billion in 2004. That's four and a half times the amount spent in 1990.

The question is, are we healthier for it? Are these new drugs really improvements over older versions? While we hear daily of new drug miracles, more often, it's the latest debacle: Baycol, a drug for lowering cholesterol, withdrawn because of deaths and transplants due to severe liver damage; Vioxx, for arthritis, withdrawn because of heart disease-related complications; and hormones such as Prempro, once seen as a boon to all post-menopausal womankind, now viewed as posing an unacceptable risk of breast cancer and heart attack.

How can this happen? As physicians, we take the Hippocratic oath to "first, do no harm." This means we pledge not to hurt our patients in any way, including by the treatments we recommend. But here is a staggering figure: almost every single prescription is in some way harmful. Just look at the warnings that come with each drug! So, if you're going to use a medication, be sure it is the right one for the purpose, use it properly, and do what you can to minimize risks of adverse side effects.

Among the most ignored side effects, which is quite common and can even be life threatening, is *nutrient depletion*. That is, most medications will rob your body of essential nutrients.

WHY I WROTE THIS BOOK

As a doctor who prescribes both medications and nutrients, I was compelled to write this book after seeing case after case of nutrient loss in patients due to prescribed medication. Neither the patient nor their doctors were aware of the cause of the increasing symptoms. Rather, the person was told that "it's part of the illness," and/or was given an additional drug or two to deal with the new symptoms. My patient Kathy's case is a perfect example of what I mean.

A fifty-seven-year-old retired schoolteacher, Kathy was being treated by her internist with the thiazide diuretic, Diuril, for high blood pressure; with Fosamax for osteoporosis; and with the beta blocker, Tenormin, for heart palpitations. She was referred to me, a psychiatrist, because she was tired, nervous, and depressed, and was having trouble sleeping. I could find no obvious psychological explanation for these symptoms, except maybe for the stress of her physical illness. The most likely common cause of her symptoms was the drugs themselves. Rather than adding an antidepressant, I checked out the known nutrient depletions caused by these drugs, did some lab testing, and came up with the following:

Kathy's tests revealed that she was deficient in several minerals—magnesium, potassium, and zinc. This could be due to any of the three medications. Low potassium and magnesium are both known to cause irregular heartbeats and high blood pressure. Fosamax can also deplete magnesium. And these depletions can cause fatigue and depression. I spoke to her internist, and he agreed to my supervising her nutritional regimen, while he oversaw the medications.

By taking daily doses of magnesium, zinc, and potassium, in addition to a high-potency multivitamin, Kathy soon overcame her symptoms. Her energy and mood came back up, and we avoided having to add an antidepressant to the mix. Once her mineral levels were restored, she was able to take lower doses of the drugs, as well. I see cases similar to Kathy's all the time, with simple solutions to what appear to be complex conditions, and where part of the problem stems from the prescribed medications themselves.

In *Supplement Your Prescription*, I'm addressing those of you who are already taking prescription drugs, to help you use them wisely. You may be a relative or other caregiver who is in charge of administering the medication, and you want to do the best for your loved one (or charge), rather than contributing unknowingly to making their condition worse. By learning about drug side effects and nutrient depletions, you'll have the tools to best approach the issue, whether treating yourself or someone else.

WHAT YOU CAN EXPECT TO LEARN

The initial chapters of this book will start with the basics:

- Chapter 1, "What You Should Know about Drugs and How They Deplete Nutrients," explains what medications really are, and how they can affect the ways in which your body absorbs and uses nutrients.

- Chapter 2, "You Hold the Keys to Your Health—Even If You Need Prescriptions," describes what nutrients are and provides the big picture of the ways in which poor diet, environmental toxins, and lifestyle choices can set the stage for nutrient depletion, with or without medications. It also notes the consequences of these depletions, and explores how getting all the right nutrients will enhance your overall health.

- Chapters 3 through 7 go into specifics, addressing specific conditions and individual drugs used to treat them, and how they affect nutrient balance. Each of these chapters will give you detailed advice about other choices you can make that enhance your biochemical balance. Drugs for diabetes, high blood pressure, high cholesterol, acid reflux, heartburn, constipation, arthritis, and depression are covered in detail.

- In Chapter 8, "Less Commonly Used Prescriptions," you'll get important information about depletions related to less commonly used medicines, including drugs for obesity, epilepsy, AIDS, contraception, menopausal symptoms, schizophrenia/bipolar disorder, gout, and cancer.

- The final chapter covers *polypharmacy* (taking multiple drugs) with some general principles to help you optimize your prescription use. Finally, you'll be given resources for accessing more information on your own.

A FRESH PERSPECTIVE ON HEALTH AND HEALING

If a warning light on your car's dashboard goes on, what do you do?

1. Unplug it so it stops flashing.

2. Pop the hood to see what's wrong, and/or take it to a mechanic.

Of course, you'd choose the second option. Better to attack the problem at its source and fix it so that your car runs smoothly. But your doctor has been trained, as I was, to address the problem—your symptoms—with a solution: a prescription. If it's an acute infection, an antibiotic may be just the right thing. On the other hand, if it's chronic heartburn, high blood sugar, elevated cholesterol, or headaches, would not you want to solve the problem at the root cause?

In my practice, I do go under the hood, and work with patients to get to the bottom of their discomfort and find the most effective, lasting solution. Even though my specialty is psychiatry, my medical training, and license to practice, includes general medicine. Your brain is an organ, and most often, any condition affecting the brain, such as low blood sugar or poor circulation, also affects the rest of the body. As a result, I wind up attending to all the health issues that I can handle appropriately. I also talk to the patient's other physicians, to be sure that we're all on the same page, and not working at cross-purposes. You deserve to have the best team that medicine has to offer.

Rather than a brief twenty-minute visit, where the doctor interrupts about every twenty seconds (as shown by research), I spend an hour and a half on the first visit, and I look for root causes, not just a quick fix. That takes time, and knowledge—biochemistry, physiology, and all the complex interactions of the various symptoms. Medical detective work, including specific lab testing, helps uncover those root causes. Only then can I determine the best treatment.

My patient Alexandra is a good case in point. A forty-eight-year-old wife and mother, she came to see me with a variety of health issues: she was taking Prozac, and was experiencing several of its side effects. Her doctor added two more medications, but she was only getting worse. Soon after seeing me, however, her condition turned around and the story had a happy ending. This is discussed in more detail in Chapter 7 on depression.

How was this case different? Instead of sending her to an endocrinologist, gynecologist, and nutritionist, I did the whole job myself. I found that her depression was due to hormone and nutrient imbalances, and not an antidepressant deficiency.

The lesson here is that your body is not segmented. It operates as a fine-tuned interplay among various systems. Treatment should address the deepest root cause, and be as safe and natural as possible. Medication doses should be kept at the lowest effective dose, which will greatly decrease or eliminate side effects.

You might ask: Why doesn't my doctor know this? Read on for the answers to how doctors are educated about drugs (and *not* educated about nutrition), and how research bias and marketing tactics of the pharmaceutical industry affect your doctor's choices.

GENERIC AND BRAND NAMES FOR DRUGS

You will notice that most of the drugs described in this book have both a generic chemical name and one or more brand names. For example, Mevacor is the brand name of the cholesterol-lowering drug lovastatin. A generic drug will go only by its generic name. The availability of generics (which cost far less than branded versions) depends upon the length of time a drug has been on the market. Current laws allow drug makers to hold sole rights to sell a new drug for twenty years, after which generics can be made and sold at much lower prices. When Mevacor has been on the market long enough to lose its patent protection, generic drug makers can manufacture the same chemical substance and sell it for far less than branded Mevacor. Assuming that the drugs are manufactured by a reputable company, the generic and brand-name drugs are identical to one another chemically. Asking for a generic version will save you and the health-care system money.

IF YOU DO CHOOSE TO STOP TAKING A DRUG, DO SO RESPONSIBLY

I don't advocate ever just stopping your prescriptions without consulting with your doctor. I do, however, recommend natural solutions to the underlying cause of your problems, which in many cases will allow you—with the help of your doctor—to reduce the number or dosages of prescriptions you are taking.

ONE

What You Should Know about Drugs and How They Deplete Nutrients

In modern times, high-tech drugs and procedures exist for most conditions, but this wasn't always so. Let's turn back the clock to see just how modern pharmaceuticals were developed.

Although we don't exactly know when human beings began to use plants for healing, we do know that many animals in the wild instinctively use plants for their own healing. Primitive human beings followed suit. Native, traditional healers throughout history have made use of nature's gifts in their efforts to preserve life and ease suffering. Over the centuries, careful observation, curiosity, and urge to study the world yielded a broad range of natural medical treatments. It turns out that many of our modern medicines are derived from traditional herbal medicines:

- Chinese and Greek pharmacies used roots from the plant *Rauwolfia serpentina*, which contains a tranquilizing substance called reserpine, now used to make drugs that treat high blood pressure.

- Foxglove leaves, once prescribed to treat heart failure, are the source of the modern heart drug, digitalis.

- Senna, a common ingredient in modern-day laxatives, can be found in ancient Middle East hieroglyphics, showing it as a treatment for constipation.

- Willow bark, the predecessor of modern aspirin, was also used medicinally in the ancient Middle East.

All over the planet, wherever humans lived, knowledge about healing plants has been passed down from generation to generation and from healer to apprentice, with that knowledge being continually refined.

THE ADVENT OF MODERN PHARMACEUTICALS

Many ancient plant medicines have been chemically altered in drug company laboratories in hopes of creating something that has a targeted, specific action when taken as a drug. This process also assures its ability to be patented, so that it will he profitable.

The key invention that enabled science to make this leap was the microscope, which was created in the nineteenth century. With this tool, scientists could see the workings of individual cells. This insight was the gateway to creating drugs that could influence specific aspects of cell function. Scientists found that specific *receptors* on cells, first seen through the microscope, act as docking points for "chemical messengers"—including natural chemicals like hormones, neurotransmitters, or chemicals from herbs and foods. Synthetic chemicals like drugs were also found to dock at these receptors. When any of these chemicals attaches to a cell receptor, it "flips a switch" in the cell, changing its function in some way.

A whole new theory of health and disease arose from these discoveries, as did a whole new way of developing drugs. Gone were the days of trial and error; foraging for medicinal plants in the woods seemed entirely too primitive compared with what replaced it: white-coated scientists leaning over microscopes, determining the effect of individual chemicals on cells and then making those substances into drugs. Pharmaceutical chemists figured out ways to tinker with natural molecules to change their absorption into the body or the way they affected individual cells, targeting them to act on specific receptors.

The era of modern pharmacology had begun.

Today, substances that show promise in technological testing are then transformed into drugs, which are then tested on animals for safety, and on humans for safety and effectiveness. A few hundred million dollars later, the drug is ready for Food and Drug Administration (FDA) approval or rejection.

This new way of creating drugs and of using them against disease was a huge departure from past medical traditions, and it became the foundation for modern *allopathic* medicine.

Why the history lesson? It's designed to help you to understand how

Allopathic Medicine

Allo means opposite; *path* means disease. According to the *American Heritage Medical Dictionary*, allopathy is "a method of treating disease with remedies that produce effects antagonistic to those caused by the disease itself."

these chemicals known as prescription and over-the-counter (OTC) drugs work, and how they can reduce your body's ability to absorb, assimilate, and utilize the nutrients in your diet.

THE DOUBLE-EDGED SWORD OF DRUG SPECIFICITY

Over the decades since pharmaceuticals went high-tech, drugs have tended to become more and more *specific*—targeted to affect a single activity in the body, with as little effect as possible on other activities.

Drugs do not "correct imbalances" or nudge a malfunctioning body system back to its perfect function. (One possible exception is when hormones are given to someone who has a hormone deficiency.) Drugs are not magic bullets; they're rough tools that have to be used carefully, with respect for their potential to *create* imbalances. It's just not possible to target a single reaction in the body without tipping others into imbalance. No matter how specific a drug is designed to be, it will have effects that go beyond its intended actions. This leads to side effects, including that of robbing the body of important nutrients.

While there is plenty of published literature about this issue (as you will see), doctors aren't taught much about nutrition, drug-nutrient depletion, and the need to prescribe specific nutrients to restore healthy function. The information appears in the medical journals, but doctors are limited in what they have time to read, have little time per patient, and have had almost no training at all in nutrition in medical school. As a result, your doctor is unlikely to instruct you to supplement the prescription that he or she is handing you.

PHARMACEUTICALS TODAY: GOOD, BUT NOT PERFECT

Before the mid-1990s, consumers had enormous faith in the miracles of modern medicine. Most of those miracles, they thought, could be found in the pills, potions, ointments, and shots made by drug companies and dispensed by pharmacies.

High cholesterol? Don't want to subsist on vegetables and oat bran? Here, take this cholesterol-lowering pill. Heartburn? Want to keep eating cheese fries three times a week? Try this acid-reducing drug for instant relief! The heartbreak of psoriasis? Here, we've got something that'll clear that right up, no problem. Feeling blue? Try this antidepressant—it's so safe, they should put it in the water!

Fast-forward to the present. Drug companies are getting a lot of bad press these days. They're accused of placing profit over people and cranking out products that are not as safe or effective as the direct-to-consumer advertisements would suggest.

They encourage you to "just ask your doctor" about taking an antidepressant to cheer you up, or a sedative to help you sleep, followed by a rapid-fire list of side effects. In her scathing book, *The Truth about the Drug Companies: How They Deceive Us and What to Do about It* (Random House, 2004), Marcia Angell, M.D., former editor of the prestigious *New England Journal of Medicine*, describes how pharmaceutical-company-sponsored research published in medical journals is actually quite biased in their favor—and not focused on the consumers' best interests at all.

Similarly, in *Overdosed America* (Harper Perennial, 2005), John Abramson, M.D., an award-winning family doctor and member of the clinical faculty at Harvard Medical School, makes the point that we are using prescriptions far too often—and more for the benefit of the drug companies' bottom-line than for our good health.

Dr. Abramson doesn't stop there. He explains that the real scientific evidence shows that many of the actions you can take to protect and preserve your own health may be far more effective than what drugs can do for you—which is why the pharmaceutical companies work so hard to keep this information under wraps. Both Angell's and Abramson's books reveal how the information that doctors rely upon to guide their treatment of common health problems, from heart disease to stroke, osteoporosis, diabetes, and arthritis, is highly skewed to maximize sales and minimize information about risks.

At best, these drugs don't live up to drug companies' promises; at worst, they have side effects severe enough to cause death. A study published in the *Journal of the American Medical Association* indicated that over 106,000 deaths occur each year due to drugs taken correctly, as prescribed, making it the fourth leading cause of death in the United States.

This figure is dwarfed by other estimates of the overall damage done by prescription drugs *outside* of hospitals: in 2003, according to the Centers for Disease Control and Prevention (CDC), there were 1.7 million emergency room visits attributable to adverse effects of medical treatments (including drugs) and surgical treatments. More than a dozen drugs that were given the FDA's stamp of approval then turned out to have dangers that led to their withdrawal. In many instances, these drugs were blockbusters that were used by millions of people all over the world, and that may have been responsible for tens of thousands of deaths. Some of these problems went undetected or didn't seem clini-cally significant in research studies, which usually involve only a few hundred to a few thousand people. Even though they are responsible for knowing this information, doctors are not always well educated about specific risks.

Let's use the drug Vioxx as an example. You might know that this anti-inflammatory pain medicine was removed from the market in 2004 because studies found an unacceptable increase in risk of heart prob-lems. In its short lifetime as a blockbuster drug, it's believed that some 20 million Americans used it at some point to treat pain, usually from arthritis. A one percent increase in risk for heart attack and stroke in users of this medicine led safety officials at the FDA to calculate that about 55,000 people may have died from heart attacks and strokes as a direct result of their use of Vioxx. Because so many people take prescrip-tion medications, these risks reach critical masses—numbering enough people to capture the eye of the media and the medical community.

The silver lining about the Vioxx debacle (not to mention the ones involving Prempro, Baycol, and several other drugs) is that it raised public consciousness about the fact that prescription drugs can have risks. Any drug powerful enough to have substantial effects on a disease process will be powerful enough to cause harm.

Potential sources of conflict of interest that might allow dangerous drugs to hit the marketplace and be marketed to billions of consumers are getting more media attention. The FDA is making new rulings to eliminate conflicts of interest between doctors who work for the FDA and get paid by drug companies to research and promote their products. Consumers are also becoming more active in researching the drugs their doctors prescribe and working with their medical teams to make edu-cated decisions about what to take—or not. (One source for checking out a drug is the manufacturer's website, which includes full disclosure of all side effects. Information on nutrient depletions can often be found on those sites as well. See the Resources section at the end of the book for other useful sites.)

Pharmaceutical companies are facing new federal limitations on the use of many of their relied-upon sales tactics. Doctors are becoming more wary of drug-company "generosity," which is often designed to encourage them to prescribe that company's products over others that might be a better fit for patients. The FDA is cracking down on drug companies who make misleading statements in TV, print, and web advertisements. Clearer labeling and package inserts are being required by the FDA to help consumers better understand that the drugs they use have risks, benefits, and potential for interactions with one another. For example, the makers of certain antidepressants have been ordered to place "black box" warnings on labels, warning of potential for suicidal thinking in children and teenagers who take those drugs.

Still, despite all the bad news that's hit the media about pharmaceuticals, the public's use of them has continued to rise at a rapid clip. It's clear that some people really do require medicines for survival. Others find that they depend on medications to help them live normal, active, joyful lives. Rest assured that your chances of being killed by an FDA-approved prescription are actually relatively small. But your chances of having more subtle side effects are much higher. When it comes to living the best life you can live, even subtle side effects can cramp your style in a big way.

You can use your medicines as a part of your overall plan for improving your life and your health—as long as you are an educated consumer of those medicines. Reading this book will increase your smarts dramatically in this regard.

DOSING ISSUES: ONE SIZE DOESN'T FIT ALL

Because most drugs today are marketed and prescribed in one-size-fits-all, standard doses, a ninety-year-old, hundred-pound grandmother on five medications is getting the same dose as a two-hundred-thirty-pound football player.

The common, one-size-fits-all drug dose ignores our biological individuality, which is influenced by gender, race, body size, individual genetics, variations in nutritional status, and other factors. For example, women generally require lower doses than men and may suffer serious side effects when given larger, man-sized doses. In 2001, the U.S. General Accounting Office (GAO) reported that in early drug studies for establishing drug doses, 78 percent of the subjects were men. No wonder so many women cannot tolerate standard doses of top-selling drugs!

Thanks to such crusaders as Jay S. Cohen, M.D., the public and the medical community are becoming aware of this issue. Dr. Cohen's book, *Over Dose: The Case Against the Drug Companies* (Tarcher/Putnam, 2001), received a glowing review in the *Journal of the American Medical Association*. In it, Dr. Cohen explains that most side effects are dose-related, and that the standard starting doses of many top-selling drugs are too strong for millions of patients. I have found this to be true in my own practice, and recommend that medications should always be started at the lowest possible dose and built up gradually. This allows you to observe both how you respond, in a positive way, and how well you are able tolerate the drug.

Another problem involves the mystery of interactions. Medical science doesn't always know how drugs will interact with each other in a patient's body. For example, a patient might simultaneously be put on Lipitor for cholesterol lowering, prednisone for respiratory relief, and Motrin for pain. How many of the health problems that crop up in this patient are *caused* by drug side effects and interactions? We just don't know, since we have no long-term studies on this.

What I have seen is that patients that have been on multiple drugs over long periods of time often show an overall deterioration in their health. Not surprising, for two reasons: 1) the drugs are gradually depleting the patient's nutrient levels, and 2) the source of the health problems have not been addressed—the drugs are only treating the symptoms. That being said, your pharmacist, besides your doctor, is an excellent resource in this regard.

AN INTRODUCTION TO DRUG-INDUCED NUTRIENT DEPLETION

Supplement Your Prescription will, in particular, educate you about a lesser-known side effect of the most commonly used medicines: the many ways in using one or more of them can rob your body's supplies of nutrients that are essential to your health.

This side effect, which is an issue with a surprising number of the most oft-prescribed drugs, doesn't hit the headlines too often; it's usually not dramatic or immediately noticeable. But over months to years of taking one or more prescription drugs every day, nutrient depletion can take a toll on your health and increase your risk of becoming ill—in some cases, with the very illness you're trying to prevent with the medication.

Many people who are depleted due to prescription drugs may think their mounting health problems are just part of aging. The consequences of drug-induced nutrient depletion can lead to the use of more and more medications—which only makes the matter worse. Couple this with the same standard American dietary and lifestyle choices that can cause the chronic conditions that create the need for drugs in the first place, and you have a potent combination of factors that can make your medications a very real detriment to your health.

Every person who takes prescription drugs needs to know about drug-induced nutrient depletion, and about how to effectively balance this side effect with appropriate nutrition from foods and supplements.

In this book, I deal primarily with drugs intended for long-term use that cause slow depletion over time with serious effects—ones that mainstream medicine rarely traces back to the medication. In fact, the allopathic game plan usually entails *adding* more drugs to counter what is really attributable to drug-induced nutrient depletion.

A DEEPER LOOK AT HOW DRUGS CAN DEPLETE NUTRIENTS

When drugs deplete your body's nutrient levels, they are likely to do so in one or more of five ways. They can:

1. Decrease appetite or increase your appetite for unhealthy foods.

2. Reduce the absorption of nutrients in the gastrointestinal (GI) tract.

3. Increase the rate at which the body breaks down a nutrient.

4. Block the action or formation of nutrients at the level of individual cells.

5. Increase the amount of nutrient flushed out of the body through the kidneys.

Here are a few examples of each kind of nutrient depletion, and how they happen:

1. *Decreased appetite, or increased appetite, for unhealthy foods that cause weight gain and replace healthy foods.* Many drugs can reduce your intake of beneficial nutrients by reducing your appetite, as with the stimulant drug Ritalin (methylphenidate), often prescribed for children. Some antidepressant drugs also tend to reduce food intake. On the flip side, a drug can reduce your nutritional status by increasing your appetite for unhealthy foods and causing you to gain weight, but without good nourishment. This can happen with some hormonal contraceptives, with some antidepressants and antipsychotics, and with any drug that includes steroids, such as prednisone (usually taken orally) and inhaled steroids used to treat asthma.

2. *Reduced absorption of nutrients.* Most drugs discussed in this book are taken by mouth. In passing through the gastrointestinal tract, they can bind to specific nutrients before they're able to be absorbed into your bloodstream.

Antibiotics can have this effect; so can weight-loss drugs and cholesterol-lowering medicines that prevent fat or cholesterol from being absorbed into the body. Drugs used to treat acid reflux or heartburn can change the environment of the GI tract in a way that reduces absorption of needed vitamins and minerals.

> **Gastrointestinal (GI) Tract**
>
> The path traveled by any solid food or drug you swallow. Includes the mouth, esophagus, stomach, small intestine, large intestine (colon), and rectum.

3. *Increased "burning" of nutrients.* Nutrients are essential to the metabolic activities of every cell in your body. They are used up in the process and replaced by new nutrients that you take in as food or supplements. Some drugs deplete nutrients by speeding up the rate at which this occurs, examples being antibiotics (including penicillin and gentamicin), and steroid drugs like prednisone and colchicine (used to treat gout).

4. *Blocking of nutrients' effects or production at the cellular level.* If you swallow your medication (as opposed to inhaling it, injecting it, or applying it to skin or mucous membranes), it's broken down in your gastrointestinal tract, just like the food you eat. It is then absorbed into tiny blood vessels (capillaries) that line your intestines, and ends up in a large vein that carries that blood to the liver. Here it's broken down by enzymes into harmless end products. The newly altered drug molecules pass out of the liver and are eventually distributed by the circulation throughout the body, where it does its job.

Because much of the drug is neutralized during this process, a much higher dose of drug may be necessary when it's taken orally than when it's absorbed through other routes. In other words, if you swallow a pill, you have to take a much higher dose than if you have the same drug injected.

Most drugs work on individual cells by interacting with receptors on their surface, or by affecting the activity of enzymes that regulate the operations of cells. It's here that some nutrients are depleted by medications through what's known as an *anti-nutrient* effect.

The medication has its intended effect on enzymes or receptors, but it also affects enzymes or receptors that are needed to process essential nutrients. For example, widely prescribed statin drugs, such as Crestor and Lipitor, block the activity of an enzyme that creates cholesterol in the body—but this action depletes the body of a substance called coenzyme Q_{10}, which is vital for heart health.

> **Enzyme**
>
> A protein that accelerates the rate of chemical reactions, without being damaged or changed by the reactions.

5. *Increased loss of nutrients through the urinary system.* Any drug that causes an increase in urination can drain the body's levels of water-soluble nutrients, including B vitamins and minerals such as magnesium and potassium. The major offenders here are drugs used to treat hypertension, particularly the diuretics that reduce blood pressure by flushing more water out of the body.

OTHER FACTORS THAT CAN CONTRIBUTE TO DRUG-NUTRIENT DEPLETION

Traits both inborn and acquired can raise your chances of becoming nutrient-depleted due to the medications you take. For example:

- Being under chronic or intense stress, either physically or mentally. This can speed up your body's "burning" of needed nutrients.

- Having a chronic disease that depletes nutrients. Many disorders fit this description. If you aren't sure whether your disease is a nutrient-robber, you can find out in the chapters on individual drugs and the conditions they are prescribed to treat.

- Having pre-existing GI problems that reduce your ability to absorb nutrients. For example: inadequate stomach acid is a common problem in older people, and this can reduce absorption of important nutrients. More on this topic in Chapter 6.

- Poor function of your liver or kidneys. If either of the body's main cleansing systems is not working well, nutrients can't be utilized properly.

- Genetic makeup that causes your body to process drugs slowly or differently than the general population, or requires more of certain nutrients. This isn't under your control, but in the near future, there may be ways to test widely for these genetic variations and to pre-scribe medicines and supplements accordingly.

- Alcohol abuse or use of recreational drugs. Using alcohol or illegal drugs along with prescriptions is dangerous. This practice can not only deplete your body of nutrients, but also an accidental overdose or a bad combination of medicines with recreational drugs and/or alcohol can be deadly!

- The use of multiple medications. Polypharmacy is a fact of life for some people, but they need to be aware that nutrient depletion can be amplified by this.

- Poor diet. This is pretty obvious. If you're eating poorly *and* taking one or more medications that deplete nutrients, you're digging a hole for yourself faster than if you're eating well and taking those same medications.

The more of these factors that ring true for you, the more likely you are to benefit from careful, targeted nutrient supplementation along with the medicines you take.

In the next chapter, I'll explain what exactly I mean when I refer to "appropriate nutritional and lifestyle changes." You'll learn what nutrients are and why some are so essential for your good health. Once you have that knowledge under your belt, you can move into the rest of the book with a solid understanding of the basics of a good nutrition and multivitamin/mineral program, and of how other lifestyle factors—stress control, exercise—fit into the big picture of your health.

TWO

You Hold the Keys to Your Health—Even If You Need Prescriptions

Whether you fall into the category of "I know what I should be eating, I'm just not doing it," or of "I like my regular American food just fine, thanks," or simply of "I don't know what I'm supposed to be eating—there's too much conflicting information out there," you're not alone.

When the United States Department of Agriculture (USDA) did a survey to see how many Americans were eating their fruit and vegetables, they found that most of us fall far short of the recommended five to seven servings a day. About 9,000 people recorded the foods they ate over a twenty-four hour span—and the results of those surveys showed that only 11 percent had eaten adequate servings of fruits and vegetables. Another large government survey, this one from the Centers for Disease Control and Prevention (CDC), found that only 23 percent of American adults meet current recommendations for exercise. (For more details on this survey, see www.cdc.gov/nchs/data/series/sr_10/sr10_232.pdf.)

Obviously, we have room for improvement in both the way we eat and our commitment to exercise. In this chapter, I'll give you some pointers on how to make these improvements in your own life—small improvements that can make a huge difference in your health.

FOOD, GLORIOUS FOOD

Think of food as fuel. In order to function at peak efficiency, your body needs the best raw material possible. Our standard American diet (SAD for short!), which emphasizes high-fat, high-calorie, low-nutrient eating, is anything but nourishing. We live in a time when food is more plentiful than it has ever been in history, yet we are woefully undernourished because we fill up on all the wrong foods.

Many of us eat too many processed foods that have almost no nutritional value. These foods are high in chemicals, salt, and, above all, sugar. Most people's bodies can't fulfill their basic nutritional needs on a diet of foods like these. In fact, modern medical minds almost all agree that all adults should take a multivitamin every day because our diets so often fall short.

Depressed, tired, foggy-brained individuals are often told by their doctors that they need an antidepressant. All many of them really need is a steady supply of real food to get their brains and bodies back on track. This has been the experience of so many of my grateful patients as they learn to use food as medicine.

Think back on the times you found yourself feeling tired, irritable, unable to think straight, and overwhelmed with all that you had to do . . . and then, you realized that you'd skipped a meal. Within minutes of eating a tuna sandwich, some cheese and crackers, or even just an apple, everything changes—the world becomes a better place, and those tasks are no longer insurmountable. The problem was low blood sugar: your poor brain was running on empty!

Low blood sugar goes away whether you eat junk food or healthy food, but long term, a diet that's low in vitamins, minerals, and other nutrients will make you tired, irritable, and absentminded. Your daily food choices make a big difference in your life, especially when you take medications that deplete nutrients.

Science has proven that following the principles of optimum nutrition can:

- Improve your mood.

- Increase your mental and physical stamina and your overall health.

- Enhance your concentration, memory, and overall mental ability.

- Reduce your stress level.

Really, your diet is the bottom-line. When you start out with long-term nutrient depletions caused by years of food choices that just don't serve your body's needs, you may already be experiencing subtle symptoms of *subclinical nutrient deficiency* or general, long-term nutritional imbalances. This can happen long before you swallow your first dose of nutrient-depleting medication.

These imbalances can contribute strongly to issues like hypertension (high blood pressure), high cholesterol, arthritis, difficult menopause, or depression. Once these conditions appear, off you trot to the doc for your prescriptions, and the medicines may well end up further depleting your body of nutrients, making you even sicker!

The information in this chapter is designed to give you the simple, basic information you need to choose a better way of eating. It's far easier to make those healthy choices once you have a good grasp of basic nutrition. In this chapter, we'll be looking at each of the various nutrients, including the fuel-supplying carbohydrates, the building-block proteins and fats, and the catalysts and cofactors, otherwise known as vitamins and minerals. We'll finish with a list of the basics that will get you—and keep you—in vibrant health.

I also hope to inspire you to get started with a basic, well-rounded supplement program to provide a rock-solid nutritional foundation. Then, as you read later chapters on individual drugs, you can fine-tune your program.

MACRONUTRIENTS: WHAT YOU NEED TO KNOW

Macronutrients (*macro* = large) are the "building blocks" of food. These include:

1. Carbohydrates that can be "burned" for energy

2. Protein that can be used to build tissues, including muscle, connective tissue, bone, and internal organs

3. Fat that can be burned for energy or stored for use as energy fuel

All foods fall into one of three categories: carbohydrate, protein, or fat. Our bodies need high-quality versions of all three for optimal health. An excellent dietary mix is to obtain about 40 percent of your calories from carbohydrates, 30 percent from protein, and 30 percent from fat.

Not all carbohydrates, protein, and fats are created equal; different foods contain different kinds of these macronutrients, and some are very good for you while others are far less so.

Running on Carbohydrates

Your body's main fuel is glucose, the simplest form of sugar and the form of carbohydrate that floats around in your bloodstream and is "burned" in the cells to make energy. Most carbohydrates—bread, cereals, fruits, and vegetables—break down into this simple sugar during digestion.

This does not mean that you should eat more sugar to enhance your energy! Quite the opposite. The quick-release sugars—found in white flour, candy, cookies, and fruit juices—will lead only to the "sugar blues." Instead, eat *complex* carbohydrates—found in whole grains, legumes, vegetables, and fruit—which release their glucose slowly over time. This gives your body the glucose it needs for fuel without the blood sugar spikes that leave you feeling tired, cranky, and craving sweets.

Adding a food rich in protein to a meal or snack will slow the release of sugars from carbohydrate-rich foods. For example, pair a couple of slices of roasted turkey with a piece of whole-grain bread, or try poached salmon with a serving of brown rice. For more information on sugar and carbs, see Nancy Appleton's classic book *Lick the Sugar Habit* (Avery, 2001).

The rate at which some carbohydrate foods break down into sugar may surprise you. Did you know that a potato turns into glucose in your body far faster than a slice of whole wheat bread? Or that carrots and bananas turn into glucose nearly as fast as a cookie does? We can measure the effect of carbohydrate-rich foods on blood sugar on a scale called the *glycemic index* (GI). Pure glucose has a GI of 100; carbohydrate sources that break down very slowly, such as lentils, can have a GI below 10. To reduce the "sugar blues," eat foods with GI of 50 or lower, and if you do eat high-GI foods (examples: white bread, baked potato, white rice), eat them with protein-rich foods, like chicken or plain yogurt.

Glycemic load (GL) is another measurement of the effect of carbohydrate-rich foods on blood sugar levels. Where GI measures one food's effect, regardless of serving size, GL measures the effect of a food *per serving*. For example: watermelon has a high GI, but because a serving of watermelon is mostly water, its GL is low.

For a more detailed ranking of which carbs are broken down most slowly, with extensive lists of foods with their GI and GL values, see www.diabetes.about.com/library/mendosagi/ngilists.htm.

Powered by Protein

Protein is made up of components called *amino acids*. It is the building block of all of the body's components, from hair and muscles to enzymes, hormones, and neurotransmitters. Eating protein can boost your metabolism by 25 percent, which really helps to burn the extra fat you've been wishing away in the mirror. Some amino acids are essential, which means we have to get them in the foods we eat; others can be created in the body from other amino acids. Meat, fish, poultry, cheese, milk, and eggs are considered *complete* proteins, because they contain the essential amino acids in a good balance. You need about 20 grams of protein per meal, which is equal to three eggs; 3 to 4 ounces of lean meat, poultry, or fish; or half a can (3 ounces) of tuna.

Dairy products, preferably organic and free of antibiotics or hormones, are also a good source of protein. Three small containers (16 ounces total) of unsweetened yogurt or a cup of cottage cheese provide all you need per meal. For vegetarians, soy hot dogs and burgers, 5 ounces of tofu, or a serving of soy-based protein powder can give you the amount of protein needed per meal. Vegetarians need to be conscientious about combining grains, beans, rice, nuts, and seeds to keep their protein intake balanced. For detailed information about the protein content of commonly eaten foods, refer to the Harvard School of Public Health's website at www.hsph.harvard.edu/nutritionsource/protein.html, or purchase Annette B. Natow and Jo-Ann Heslin's book *The Protein Counter* (Pocket Books, 2003).

Fats Are Essential

Contrary to popular belief, fats don't make you fat. In fact, certain fats are essential in keeping your body healthy. Just as proteins are built from amino acids, fats are built from *fatty acids*. Some fatty acids are extremely beneficial to your health while others are best avoided.

Over the past twenty years, the low-fat diet craze has caused many people to replace fat in their diets with low-fat carbohydrates, and the result has been a nationwide epidemic of obesity. Imbalanced or inadequate intake of fats can cause everything from PMS and infertility to depression, anxiety, and even premature aging. Research conducted at Harvard showed that high-carbohydrate, low-fat diets may actually increase the risk of heart disease by reducing the levels of the protective or "good" HDL (high-density lipoprotein) cholesterol in the bloodstream.

There is strong supporting evidence that the low-fat boom led to the current obesity trend. Just look at the numbers. According to the Center for Health Statistics, the American obesity epidemic started in the early 1980s—at the same time that the market was being flooded with low-fat products. Suddenly, the rate of overweight in adults went through the roof. At the start of the 1980s, 13 to 14 percent of adults were overweight; by the end of that decade, the rate of overweight rose to nearly 25 percent of adults.

Yes, there are "bad" fats—the trans-fatty acids found in most baked goods and many processed foods, for example. Saturated or animal fats are widely considered to be "bad" as well, but they are acceptable in moderation when eaten along with protein in meat and dairy products.

About 30 percent of the calories in your diet should come from good fats. The most healthy fatty acids are found in fish oil, flaxseed oil (both have lots of *omega-3* fatty acids), and borage oil (which has a type of omega-6 fatty acid, *gamma-linolenic acid* or GLA, that has many health benefits). These omega-3 and omega-6 fats stimulate the immune system and fight inflammation, a known cause of heart disease and many other chronic diseases. They also support optimal brain function. Fatty fish like salmon, tuna, and mackerel contain the highest concentration of omega-3s. Aside from GLA from borage oil, which is used as a supplement (oatmeal is another good source), the omega-6 fatty acids found in meat, milk, vegetable oils, seeds, and nuts are rarely scarce in the standard American diet. In fact, although we need them for good health, most of us are consuming too many.

Most of us eat about twenty times more omega-6 fatty acids than omega-3s in products like cereals, whole-grain bread, baked goods, fried foods, margarine, and others. For an adequate omega-3 supply, you should eat fatty fish three times a week or take 1,000 milligrams (mg) of omega-3 fatty acids daily as a supplement. (Use the supplement you choose according to the instructions on the label.) You can add good fats by sprinkling a heaping tablespoon of ground flaxseed on salads, cereals, or vegetables daily.

When you shop for cooking oils, olive oil is always a winner—but the fatty acids it contains won't help to boost your levels of omega-3s. To promote better omega-3/omega-6 balance in the foods you prepare with oil, seek out organic, cold-pressed seed oil blends like flaxseed, soybean, macadamia, sesame, walnut, and almond. These oils provide omega-6 and omega-3 fatty acids in the right ratio of around 2:1 to 3:1.

Why cold-pressed oils? Because the heat and chemicals used in other types of refining processes destroy the fatty acids in the oils. However, you cannot cook with most cold-pressed oils because they degrade when heated. Use them on salads, put them on baked potatoes in place of butter, or drizzle them over steamed veggies for a delicious treat. Olive oil, macadamia nut oil, and cold-pressed sesame oil can be used for cooking at low temperatures, but you may lose some of the healthiest ingredients if you attempt to use them to fry foods.

Reduce your intake of beef and pork because they are high in saturated fat. This less healthy form of fat is also likely to contain hormones, antibiotics, and pesticide residues from animals raised on factory farms. You can reduce your exposure to these chemicals—some of which are known causes of cancer—by shopping for organic meats from grass-fed cattle. (Organic, grass-fed meat is also less likely to carry mad cow disease.) Eat the leanest cuts possible. Skinless chicken and turkey are better sources of protein as they contain little saturated fat.

Eliminate trans-fatty acids from your diet. Fried foods, especially French fries, fried chicken, and doughnuts, are almost always soaked in these toxic fats. Food manufacturers have to tell you, on their labeling, how much of these fats their products contain, but you should know that a product that contains less than half a gram (0.5 grams) of trans-fatty acids per serving can be labeled as zero grams. To be safe, stay away from foods like chips, crackers, and packaged baked goods, all of which are likely to contain some amount of hydrogenated or partially hydrogenated vegetable oils—trans fats.

Eggs contain omega-3 fatty acids as well. They've been demonized because their yolks are high in cholesterol, but studies show that eating an egg or two a day won't raise your cholesterol counts. You can buy eggs from organically raised chickens that have eaten feed enriched with the omega-3 fat docosahexanoic acid (DHA) to boost your omega-3 intake by about 200 mg per egg.

EXTRACTING ENERGY FROM MACRONUTRIENTS: OXIDATION AND ANTIOXIDANTS

Once you get all that good food into your body, the work has just begun. You have to digest and absorb it, and then your cells have to transform it into: 1) building blocks for tissues; and 2) energy.

The key to energy production in the body is oxygen. Oxygen is the ultimate "essential"—a few minutes without it and, of course, we'll die. Have you ever thought about what happens to oxygen once it enters your body?

You inhale and send oxygen-rich air into your lungs. That oxygen passes into your bloodstream, and is taken up into individual cells. Those cells use it to help burn food to produce energy, in a process called *oxidation*. As cells use oxygen to metabolize (break down to create energy) carbohydrates, fat, and protein, they create a kind of "exhaust" or waste known as *free radicals*. Oxidation and free-radical formation are behind the rusting of nails and the browning of apple slices. In the body, they can do damage to the fats and proteins from which your cells are built. They can even harm DNA, the genetic blueprint that creates who you are, and are considered to underlie many conditions, including cancer, atherosclerosis, and Alzheimer's disease.

Fortunately, your body has a defense: specific nutrients that neutralize those free radicals. Fruit and vegetables, whole grains, beans, green tea, and herbs are good for you for many reasons—they're loaded with essential nutrients—but science is revealing that the value of these foods can especially be traced back to their bounty of nutrients that prevent free-radical damage: the *antioxidants*. Your body can make a lot of antioxidants on its own, but you also need the ones found in healthy foods.

Problems arise when 1) you don't consume enough antioxidant-rich foods to neutralize free radicals; 2) you take medicines that reduce your body's production of its own antioxidants; or 3) you are exposed to a lot of exhaust fumes, air pollution, cigarette smoke, or meats that have been fried, preserved with nitrates, or broiled. All of these influences cause your body to make more free radicals. High-stress living, very intense exercise regimens, or overexposure to the sun have the same effect of increasing your need for antioxidant nutrients.

This means that most people living in the modern world have high need for antioxidants—especially when you consider the fact that many commonly used drugs reduce the body's production of such antioxidants as *coenzyme Q_{10}* (depleted by statin drugs) and *glutathione* (depleted by the over-the-counter drug acetaminophen, or Tylenol).

How can you keep free radicals at bay? Increase your intake of antioxidants, a family of nutrients with the power to mop them up. Top antioxidant foods include prunes, raisins, blueberries, and blackberries, followed by kale, spinach, strawberries, raspberries, plums, broccoli, and alfalfa sprouts. You can amp up your antioxidant power even more by adding antioxidant supplements to your diet. You'll learn more about this throughout the coming chapters.

How to Eat Your Antioxidants

You can easily increase your daily intake of antioxidants and reap their rewards by following these suggestions:

- *Eat at least five servings a day of fruits and vegetables.* Studies show that this number of servings of fruits and veggies is the minimum that will protect against many diseases, including cancer, stroke, and degenerative diseases.

- *Try something new.* Enjoy all the variety in the plant kingdom—you'll get a well-rounded daily dose of natural antioxidants. Although there are 150,000 edible plant species on earth, most people limit themselves to iceberg lettuce, tomatoes, potatoes (mainly as French fries), bananas, and oranges (mainly as juice). When you eat a wide variety of these foods, you'll reap the benefits of a wide variety of plant chemicals (*phytonutrient* or *phytochemicals*), each with its own special benefits.

- *Think—rainbow colors, fresh, and unusual!* Plant chemicals known as *phytonutrients,* which are rich in antioxidant power, come in a great variety of colors. Picture a cornucopia of fruits and vegetables: crunchy orange carrots; deep purple eggplants; bright red plump tomatoes; shiny green peppers; luscious purple grapes; abundant green leaves of lettuce, kale, and spinach; yellow and green squash; large juicy peaches. These are nature's gifts, filled with an incredible array of vitamins, minerals, and phytonutrients that nourish and heal us. *The deeper the color, the more antioxidants and other beneficial phytochemicals you're getting.* These foods also are rich in fiber that aids in digestion and carbohydrates that break down slowly for steady energy. Some even contain protein. To support your movement towards a more colorful diet, refer to *Eat Your Colors* by Marcia Zimmerman, M.Ed., C.N. (Owl Books, 2001), and *What Color is Your Diet* by David Heber, M.D. (HarperCollins, 2001).

Fruits and vegetables are best bought fresh, the closer to picking time the better, and eaten soon after. Next best is frozen; canned should be your last resort. You can eat vegetables raw, steamed, or lightly sautéed in olive oil. The varieties are endless. Add healthy salad dressings—ones without sugar, MSG, and other chemicals. Or make your own with sesame oil, soy sauce, and some spices and herbs that have their own nutritional value.

Spices and Herbs

Besides adding taste to foods that might otherwise be less appealing than standard junk-food fare, herbs and seasonings are wonderful sources of antioxidants and provide missing elements in the diet. Cinnamon, cilantro, parsley, garlic, oregano, turmeric (cumin), ginger, and rosemary are just a few of the herbal superstars of the kitchen that have known healing effects.

The Salt Issue

Limit your intake of normal table salt. It is processed sodium chloride and is as bad for you as any other processed food. On the other hand, sea salt in its natural form is essential for good cellular function. It contains trace minerals, including iodine—the mineral usually added to table salt, important for the health of the thyroid gland—in a concentration that is more usable by the body.

If you crave salt, this may be a sign of low thyroid and adrenal function. Salt is particularly important for balanced function of many of the body's glands and organs. (The thyroid and adrenal glands make hormones that play roles in your energy levels and help keep you at an ideal weight; reduced function in either can lead to fatigue and weight gain.) Rather than reaching for the potato chips, though, add pure sea salt to your food, in moderation. But if your doctor has ordered a low-sodium diet for you, stick with that.

WHICH DIET IS BEST FOR YOU?

The simplest, healthy diet to follow is the *Mediterranean diet,* inspired by the traditional eating patterns of some of the Mediterranean countries such as Greece and Southern Italy. Common elements include eating generous amounts of fruits, vegetables, and whole grains; consuming fish on a regular basis; drinking red wine in moderation; using olive oil; and eating very little red meat—basically, a high-fiber, high-antioxidant, low-animal fat, high-monounsaturated fat (that's the fat in olive oil) diet.

You can effortlessly maintain good health and proper weight, and control inflammation with this diet, which contains almost no processed foods. And you can lose weight on this diet, especially if you stay away from processed breads and sugars. However, if weight loss is your goal, or you have a lot of weight to lose or serious health problems to deal with, you can just cut out the whole grains for a while, or try the Zone diet (see next page). Even though this book is about drug-nutrient depletion and not diet, I do know that many of the conditions that lead you to take prescriptions in the first place are related to poor diet and overweight. So healthy weight loss, and simply, healthy eating, should be an essential part of your program.

If you are eating the standard American diet, shifting to the Zone diet, consisting of a 40-30-30 ratio of carbohydrates, protein, and fat—will shed pounds. The program is safe and works like a charm to jump-start a lifetime of healthy eating. To learn more, see *What to Eat in the Zone* (Harper, 2003), and several others Zone books by Barry Sears, M.D.

People who badly need to lose weight, reduce cholesterol counts, stop the downward spiral of diabetes, or improve cardiovascular health can take a more intense approach. The fastest shortcut to better health and reduced body fat is to eat a diet low in carbohydrates. A favorite of mine is the "Paleolithic" or "Stone Age" diet, developed by Loren Cordain, Ph.D. Like our caveman ancestors who were hunter-gatherers, you eat meat, chicken and fish, eggs, fruit, vegetables (especially root vegetables), nuts, and berries, and avoid grains, potatoes, sugar, dairy, and salt. Anyone interested in learning more about this diet should read Dr. Cordain's book, *The Paleo Diet* (Wiley, 2002).

Other excellent diet books include Ann Louise Gittleman's *Fat Flush Plan* (McGraw-Hill, 2002) and *Fat Flush Cookbook* (McGraw-Hill, 2003). Another one filled with great recipes is Sandra Woodruff's *Secrets of Good-Carb Low Carb Living* (Avery, 2004).

MICRONUTRIENTS: VITAMINS, MINERALS, AND ANTIOXIDANTS

To achieve optimum health and nutrition, you need to "eat right *and* take a multivitamin," as a recent headline in the prestigious *New England Journal of Medicine* editorial put it. "The evidence suggests that people who take such supplements are healthier."

Like carbohydrates, protein, and fats, vitamins and minerals are essential to good health. They are considered micronutrients (*micro* = small) because they are needed in relatively small quantity compared to the macronutrients.

Vitamins and minerals function as cofactors, or chemical helpers, in the chemical processes that occur at every moment in every one of the three trillion or so cells of your body. Getting enough of these micronutrients into your body will boost many body functions, bringing broad improvements in mental and physical health. For instance:

- B vitamins can protect you from depression, anxiety, stress, confusion, fatigue, mental dullness, and emotional fragility, and can even boost your IQ.

- The minerals magnesium and calcium have hundreds of functions in your body, and promote bone health, steady heartbeat, and flexible, open blood vessels. These minerals also help improve asthma symptoms and reduce muscle cramping.

- Vitamin K promotes bone health and healthy blood clotting.

- Good micronutrient nutrition, which also includes iron, zinc, manganese, chromium, and antioxidant nutrients such as the mineral selenium and vitamins A, C, and E, bring enhanced energy, memory, blood sugar regulation, and immunity.

The *recommended daily allowance* (RDA) of essential nutrients is intended to be available entirely through food. In reality, it is impossible to get these levels through the food available to us today, because our soil has become depleted in essential nutrients. Even fresh and wholesome foods straight from the fields have lower quantities of these essential vitamins and minerals than they had fifty or one hundred years ago. More nutrients are lost in transit from farm to table.

Recent analyses of nearly a dozen popular diet plans show that none of them provide 100 percent of the RDAs for thirteen vitamins and minerals. What's more, the RDAs are a one-size-fits-all approach to nutrition, and each of us has different requirements. Individual physiology, lifestyle, stress, age, prescription drug use, and physical condition all weigh heavily on our nutritional needs. The RDA is not enough to keep us in optimal health.

Consider this research. Ninety students were assigned to one of three groups: one group received a multivitamin and mineral supplement; the second group received an identical-looking placebo (dummy pill); and the third group, nothing. After seven months, the IQ of those taking the supplements had increased by a staggering nine points! A five-point increase would get half the learning-disabled children out of special schools and back to normal schooling.

My own project, Nourish America (formerly Vitamin Relief USA), supplies more than 26,000 (soon to be 2.5 million) at-risk children around the country with daily multivitamin tablets. It has shown similar results: better health, less absenteeism, improved learning and behavior, and less aggression. We are also supplying 3,000 seniors who are at risk for malnutrition with multivitamins, and we get wonderful letters all the time, thanking us for the difference our vitamins have made in their health and well-being (www.nourishamerica.org).

Even if your diet is perfect, the world you live in isn't. We're surrounded by toxins and pollutants, some of which we take in through our food. We need extra nutrient protection to help guard against the harm they can do. Most of us have stressful, busy lives, which means higher nutrient requirements. And—let's face it—who has a perfect diet? Taking your "multi" takes the guesswork out of getting the amounts you need to avoid frank deficiency of any essential nutrient.

If you are taking medications, a multinutrient program will help give you broad protection against nutritional depletion, which you can then tailor to your specific needs as you read relevant chapters.

A BASIC SUPPLEMENT PLAN—FOR EVERY BODY

The science of micronutrients has progressed by leaps and bounds since the 1970s, when consumers first started to catch on to the idea that supplementation makes sense. We know a great deal about how nutrients interact, and about how to get the proper complement of nutrients into a daily supplement program. Let's get you started on a multi-nutrient supplement plan that will benefit every adult.

Here are guidelines on what to look for on the label of your daily multivitamin, although formulas will certainly vary, as will your own personal needs. *Most will not contain this amount in the daily dose, so supplement with extra doses.* For example, most have 400 international units (IU) of vitamin D, though recent research puts the daily requirement somewhere between 1,000 and 2,000 IU; or vitamin C at 250 milligrams (mg), while I'd recommend at least 1,000 mg daily. If your multivitamin requires that you take several tablets a day, it's best to gradually work your way up to the recommended dose.

Unless otherwise advised, take supplements with food to aid in their digestion and to prevent side effects such as nausea, often due to the B vitamins.

As you read later chapters for specific drugs and conditions, you will learn in-depth about many of the vitamins, minerals, antioxidants, and accessory nutrients listed in Table 2.1 on page 32.

I also recommend adding, daily:

- 30 mg of coenzyme Q_{10}, an antioxidant and heart health promoter (more on this nutrient in Chapter 4).

- 1 gram (1,000 mg) of fish oil, twice daily, to supply omega-3 fatty

TABLE 2.1. RECOMMENDED DAILY MULTIVITAMIN AND MINERAL FORMULA

NUTRIENT	DAILY DOSE	ABOUT THIS NUTRIENT
Vitamin A	20,000 IU, at least 10,000 of which should be mixed carotenes	Fat-soluble vitamin needed for eyes and nervous system. Carotenes are powerful antioxidants, and many can be transformed into vitamin A in the body as needed.
Vitamin B_1 (thiamine)	25 mg	Essential for many biochemical processes in the body such as nervous system function and cellular energy production. Controls levels of homocysteine, implicated in heart disease and Alzheimer's disease.
Vitamin B_2 (riboflavin)	25 mg	
Vitamin B_3 (niacin/niacinamide)	50 mg	
Vitamin B_5 (pantothenic acid)	50 mg	
Vitamin B_6 (pyridoxine)	50 mg	
Vitamin B_{12} (cyanocobalamin)	10 mcg	
Biotin	50 mcg	
Folic acid	400 mcg	
Vitamin C	250–1,000 mg	Functions as antioxidant and immune-booster; promotes gum and connective tissue health.
Vitamin D	400–2000 IU	Builds bone. Antidepressant. Anti-cancer agent.
Vitamin E	400 IU	Powerful antioxidant.
Vitamin K	80 mcg	Aids in proper blood clotting.
Calcium	1,000 mg	Builds bone, helps in transmission of nerve impulses.
Magnesium	500 mg	Balances calcium, improves bone health, and has cardiovascular benefits.
Zinc	25 mg	Immune booster.
Boron	3 mg	Needed for proper enzyme function and cellular energy production; boron is also important for bone building.
Copper	2 mg	
Iron	2 mg for premenopausal women; men and meno-pausal women don't need extra iron, unless prescribed by a physician	
Manganese	5 mg	
Potassium	99 mg	
Chromium	200 mcg	Helps balance blood sugar; especially good for diabetics.
Iodine	150 mcg	Required for proper function of the thyroid gland.
Selenium	200 mcg	Works with vitamin E to protect against oxidation.
Molybdenum	300 mcg	Needed by many of the body's enzymes.

IU = international units; mg = milligrams; mcg = micrograms

acids. (Flax oil can be substituted by strict vegetarians, but the omega-3s in flax aren't as useful to the body as those in fish oil.)

- A probiotic supplement, which contains live, "friendly" bacteria that promote good digestion and elimination (great for chronic constipation). Probiotics, literally meaning "for life," are the friendly bacteria that reside in our digestive tracts. They help us to digest our food and absorb its nutrients, manufacture vitamins A, B, and K, and maintain optimal immune function. Unfortunately, they are often destroyed by antibiotics, birth control pills, stress, alcohol, acid-blocking drugs, and infections. Use a supplement that contains at least 1 billion live bacteria per dose.

At the end of each chapter on drugs that deplete, you will find a more or less complete listing of the nutrients covered in that chapter (Exception: Chapter 8, which deals with many different drug classes.) This is meant not as a prescription, but as a guideline—a list of the possibilities for both replacing depleted nutrients and supporting your body's return to health.

Start with the foundation of the multivitamin and other core nutrients listed here, and allow yourself a few weeks to adjust and notice any differences in how you feel and function or in your requirements for medication. Add additional nutrients or herbs one at a time, keeping track of additional changes in your health—that way, you'll get a feel for what helps most. The inset "Choosing Supplements" on page 34 offers some suggestions about what to look for in a nutritional supplement.

You can safely use the vitamins, minerals, and antioxidants recommended in each chapter. The doses offered are safe and won't harm you even if you use them with your medications. When it comes to herbs and amino acids, more care is required, especially when you are taking medications. Consult with your pharmacist and physician as you work out your total supplement plan.

NUTRITION BASICS

Whether you take prescription drugs or not, your diet and supplement program provide an essential foundation of your day-to-day health and well-being. No drug can replace a diet with a proper balance of good fats, complex carbohydrates, and high-quality protein. Neither can any nutritional supplement, for that matter—they are "supplements," not food replacements. Here are the basics to keep in mind:

Choosing Supplements

As you navigate the vast supplement marketplace, you may find yourself wondering: Can I just buy the cheapest version of a nutrient or herb? Will I get what I pay for if I buy the pricier version? Why don't supplement bottles tell me what they're for—or any other information I can use to make a choice?

In terms of cost and quality, it really is "buyer beware." Many reputable, quality-conscious supplement makers strive to give you the best possible product at the lowest possible cost. Others are just trying to cash in on the popularity of nutritional supplements, putting the bare minimum of a nutrient into a supplement—or even offering less or different ingredients than stated on the product's label.

To be sure that the supplement you are buying contains what is on the label and is of high quality, buy from reputable sources. Look for a brand that uses a third-party testing program like USP—the United States Pharmacopoeia. A USP-certified supplement will have a Verified Dietary Supplement Mark on its label. This shows that the USP has tested the supplement to make sure that it:

- Contains all the listed ingredients, in the declared amounts.

- Does not contain harmful levels of contaminants.

- Will break down properly and release its ingredients in the body, instead of passing through your digestive system without dissolving.

- Has been made according to good manufacturing practices (GMP).

The USP is independent and non-profit, and its standards can be enforced by the Food and Drug Administration (FDA). You can find a list of USP-verified supplements at www.usp.org/USPVerified/dietarySupplements/supplements.html.

Also, look for supplements that have websites and an 800 number you can call with questions or concerns.

As you shop around for supplements, you may wonder why they don't have more helpful information on their labels. Labeling information is strictly limited by the Dietary Supplement Health and Education Act (DSHEA), which the FDA passed in 1994. DSHEA created new guidelines for supplement makers about how they could market, package, and label their products—and put strong limits on any claims made about the medicinal use of those products.

A supplement label can make "structure and function claims," which describe only the ways in which the nutrients affect the body's structure or function. But it can't state that the supplement prevents or treats any disease. For example, a vitamin C label can read, "Helps promote better immune system function," but it can't say, "Shortens the number of days you suffer from a cold." This is why books like this one are such important sources of information for consumers who want to use supplements safely and effectively.

When shopping for herbs, look for a version that is *standardized*. This means that it contains a specific amount of one main ingredient—the one determined by science to be the "active" ingredient. When an herb is standardized, you know that each time you take it, it has the same effect with the same strength on your body. Why not just take a pill containing *only* the active ingredient? Because the other aspects of the herb are valuable, too. They all work together, and they are all beneficial.

- Eat three servings a day of top-quality protein foods such as fish, poultry, lean meat (free range), eggs, soy, or combinations of beans, lentils, and grains.

- Avoid hydrogenated and partially hydrogenated fats, and reduce your intake of saturated fats from meat, dairy products, and junk food.

- Choose low-GI/GL complex carbohydrates such as whole grains, vegetables, and fruits, and avoid sugar and refined foods.

- Eat fish three times a week, or take fish oil supplements.

- Use cold-pressed seed oils in salad dressings.

- Drink at least two quarts (64 ounces) of water a day, either pure or in diluted juices, and herbal or fruit teas.

- Minimize your intake of tea, coffee, and alcohol.

- Eat lots of antioxidant-rich fruits and vegetables—at least five servings a day.

- Take these supplements daily: a high-potency multivitamin formula, 1–3 grams of vitamin C, 30 mg of CoQ$_{10}$, a probiotic supplement containing 1 billion live bacteria per dose, an antioxidant formula, and 1 gram of fish oil, twice daily.

EXERCISE AND SELF-CARE BASICS

You need a minimum of twenty minutes worth of exercise a day. Ideally, you'll find time to fit in about four hours worth of aerobic exercise each week—that's enough to reduce your chances of a heart attack and some cancers by 50 percent. Exercise enhances your mental processing abilities by 20 percent, and improves mood and energy.

This doesn't mean you have to spend four hours a week in an aerobics class. Start thinking of ways to incorporate movement into your life. Put an exercise bike or an aerobic step (the kind you use in step classes at the gym) in front of the TV and *move* while you watch your favorite programs. Do abdominal crunches or squats during the commercials. Use stairs instead of an elevator; do heel raises while you wait in a line; park at the far end of parking lots; meet up with a friend or friends for talking and walking, instead of sitting and drinking frappuccinos. More focused workouts are good, too: cardiovascular exercise that gets your heart rate up and your body sweaty, plus twice weekly strength training, are good options. If you think you hate to exercise, *you just haven't found the right kind of exercise yet.* Try something new.

The best exercise for you is the kind that you enjoy and look forward to.

I'm a big fan of yoga, hiking, and Pilates, but maybe you're better suited to water exercise and weight training, or maybe swing dancing, push-ups, and sit-ups are more your speed. Maybe you'd rather shoot hoops with some friends for a half-hour, or jump up and down on a mini-trampoline in front of an afternoon talk show. If you think taking long walks is boring, get yourself a portable music player and listen to tunes or a book on tape while you stride.

Yoga and Pilates are wonderful because they promote an inward focus and help you to relax and be in the moment. They help you to become more aware of your body and appreciative of its potential. Also, they enable you to carry out both aerobic and strength-building work at the same time.

As important as it is to get your heart rate up, you also need to *relax* and release stress—especially if you're a Type A personality who never stops worrying and hurrying. Your state of mind holds huge sway over your body, and when you find ways to relax and enjoy life, your body becomes healthier. Aromatherapy, time management techniques, deep breathing, meditation, spiritual observances, and creative endeavors (journaling, creative writing, painting, dance) are all wonderful outlets that will help to center and relax you.

Don't think you have to stop worrying or hurrying entirely. The trick is to train your body in ways that allow you to remain calm even as you deal with your hectic life. This is possible, even for the most Type A individual. All you need to do is seek out the right practices for you.

Relaxation just plain feels good, but it's also important for your health. Shifting your body and mind from tense and overwhelmed to relaxed and mellow causes highly health-promoting changes in hormone and neurotransmitter levels in your body.

THE POWER OF EACH CHOICE

You must have a good base in the food you eat and the supplements you take. And no medicine or supplement can make up for lack of physical activity when it comes to looking and feeling your best.

You and you alone have the power to make the right choices for yourself—the choices that shift into greater wellness: to take a walk rather than watch TV, or to eat a healthy salad instead of fast food. Take your daily multi, eat a healthy diet, and exercise daily, and you will be well on your way to good health.

Adding extra nutrients to help offset drug-induced depletions is the next step.

THREE

Prescriptions for Blood Sugar Balance: Diabetes Drugs

As forty-two-year-old Gloria walked into my office for an initial consultation, her problem was obvious: she was overweight, with a bulging belly. She said she was tired all the time, had trouble sleeping, and was craving sweets, especially in the evening.

Her family doctor had told her she was prediabetic. This meant that a test of her blood sugars had been high after a doctor-ordered overnight fast. She had high "bad" LDL (low-density lipoprotein) cholesterol, high triglycerides, and borderline high blood pressure. He had prescribed metformin for her high blood sugar, a statin drug for her cholesterol, a diuretic for her high blood pressure, and a low-fat, low-calorie diet for her weight.

His prediction was accurate: she was on her way to becoming a full-blown diabetic. However, she was concerned about medication side effects, and asked me whether there was a better, more natural approach she could try before resorting to drugs. She didn't want to go the route that her father had—long-term diabetes, many hospitalizations, and the loss of several toes to gangrene—but she wanted to try to deal with her disease using a minimum of drugs. I told her we'd work together for the best solution, which could be some combination of diet, supplements, and—possibly—medication.

Her diagnosis was metabolic syndrome, a prediabetic condition that includes insulin resistance, elevated blood sugar, excessive visceral or belly fat, and cardiovascular problems including high cholesterol and high blood pressure. In most people who don't take big steps toward healthful living, metabolic syndrome evolves into type 2 diabetes—a disease that has reached epidemic proportions worldwide. It is also known as non-insulin dependent diabetes mellitus (NIDDM), or adult-onset diabetes, but this latter term is less used today, as the number of children and teens afflicted rises year by year.

Medications administered to type 2 diabetics have strong potential to cause nutrient depletion, as you'll see. What's more, *these depletions have been found to increase the risk of two of the major complications of the disease—heart disease and stroke*. The result is that a person with diabetes can experience the added risk of a heart attack or stroke, on top of the roughly two- to three-fold increase incurred by the illness itself—*just from taking their medicines as prescribed*.

If you are a diabetic, you'll first need a detailed, thorough understanding of your condition in order to take the best care of yourself. If you are insulin resistant like Gloria, but not yet frankly diabetic—and many insulin resistant people are being given medicines to try to *prevent* the onset of type 2 diabetes—you need this information for the same reason, and for another, more pressing one. Once you grasp the full picture, you'll see that *you can stop yourself from ever developing this disease*. Even if it runs in your family, you can prevent it, or reverse its early stages, with changes in diet and exercise habits.

TYPE 2 DIABETES: WHAT IT IS, WHO'S AFFECTED

Worldwide, obesity and overweight, and the health risks that have been linked to them, are becoming as common as malnutrition and food lack, and in every age group, too. Globally, fast food, junk food, and sugary sodas and other drinks are increasingly accessible. These affordable, convenient sources of calories are being gobbled down in place of nutritious, traditional ethnic fare, and the result is weight gain . . . and ever-rising rates of type 2 diabetes.

Junk food accounts for 90 percent of diabetes diagnoses, affecting some 177 million people worldwide. Obesity, where body weight is 30 percent or more beyond ideal, is a major risk factor for diabetes.

Formerly a disease of middle age, it's now affecting our children and adolescents in increasing numbers. Almost one out of three children and teens is considered overweight, and according to the American Obesity Association, 15 percent are frankly obese. The World Health Organization (WHO) estimates that the number of diabetics worldwide will balloon to 300 million by 2025. And, according to the American Diabetes Association, about a third of people with diabetes *don't know they have it*—until symptoms become so severe that they can't ignore them any longer.

As you may already know, type 2 diabetes is a high-maintenance disease. It requires multiple medications, possibly including daily insulin injections; blood-glucose monitoring equipment; frequent doctor's visits; and, as complications mount, is likely to lead to surgeries (including open heart surgery or amputations), dialysis, and increasing disability. As you can see, this progressive condition causes damage to the body in many ways.

The good news, if caught early, diabetes can be controlled without medications. In most cases, the disease is directly attributable to the hallmarks of unhealthy living: poor diet, obesity (especially around the stomach), and lack of physical activity.

This is how I explained it to Gloria: "Here's what's happening inside your body while you sit in your chair, munching happily on your low-fat cookies, watching your favorite TV show. Those cookies are all starch and sugar, and they break down very rapidly in your stomach to glucose, the simplest form of sugar. That glucose is sucked into your bloodstream through the walls of your small intestines, causing an abrupt rise in your levels of blood sugar. You get a delicious sugar rush, and life is good!"

She nodded in agreement, with a guilty smile.

"Enter the pancreas, a small organ that's tucked away in a curve near the top of the long, winding small intestine. It pumps digestive enzymes into the small intestine, and it also makes the hormone insulin. It senses rising blood sugar. The steeper that rise, the more abrupt the pancreas's insulin response. A burst of insulin is pumped into your blood.

"Insulin has several jobs in the sugar department: First of all, it moves glucose from the bloodstream into the cells, where it can be used to make energy; it also promotes the storage of extra sugar in muscle, and of any extra calories as fat. It's both *anabolic*—tissue-building—and *catabolic*—enabling the body to burn food as fuel.

"So your insulin response kicks in to clear your blood of the cookie-induced glucose. Your blood sugar then crashes—and levels can get very low."

"That's the opposite of diabetes, right?"

"Yes . . . type 2 diabetics get *hyperglycemic*, but I'm talking about *hypoglycemia*, where you start to feel shaky and light-headed. And what do you think happens next? You start to crave your next fix of quick-burning carbohydrates. You head for the pantry again and start the cycle all over again."

"How did you know?" Gloria wondered.

I didn't know this because of my awesome psychic powers. I knew because this is the story for virtually every person who, like Gloria, eats the standard American diet. People who eat diets heavy on the sugars and processed starches have been putting their bodies through these paces several times a day for years, decades, or even for more than half a century. Weight gain is a common result.

Your energy and mood are likely to peak and drop along with this daily cycle. Eventually you're likely to start feeling exhausted most of the time, and to get a lift, drink massive amounts of coffee. And, in the worst case, your body begins to become insensitive to insulin—that's *insulin resistance*—where your blood sugar level may remain high, above healthy limits.

Eventually, your body cells start to (figuratively) say, "Enough already! You've got enough fuel stored up to last you six weeks' worth of hiking up Mount Everest. From now on, when insulin knocks, I'm not opening the door." This is insulin resistance: the beginnings of type 2 diabetes.

The pancreas sees that the cells aren't responding to its insulin knocking on the cells' doors to let the glucose enter; so, it responds by sending out more and more of insulin to knock even more loudly and persistently. At this point, some glucose will be carried into the cells, and the high blood sugar levels will come down toward normal. This is why insulin resistance can continue for some time without causing any symptoms; the insulin response rises in intensity in order to maintain more or less normal blood sugar levels. Weight gain, caused by the body's natural response to high levels of insulin, may be the only sign for a long while. You may just think that you're taking in too many calories, not getting enough exercise, and just plain getting older.

But then, after years of this effort, the pancreas poops out. It can no longer overcome insulin resistance at the cellular level. This is the point of no return, where you can be diagnosed with type 2 diabetes.

Symptoms may slowly begin to creep in: extreme thirst and hunger, skin infections, fatigue, weight loss (generally in type 1 diabetes), cuts

Dangerous Curves

Ideally, when you've been fasting overnight or for a few hours, your blood glucose levels will be between 80 and 100 milligrams per deciliter (mg/dL). After a meal, they should gently rise no higher than 139 mg/dL, with a gradual drop no lower than 65 mg/dL. A graph of the changes in your blood sugar from fasting through a meal to after the meal has been completely digested and processed—called the postprandial curve—should be a gentle curve with no abrupt rises or falls. The higher the peak of the postprandial curve, the more insulin resistant you are.

or bruises that heal too slowly, blurred vision, or tingling or numbness in hands or feet. If you are fortunate enough, like Gloria, to recognize insulin resistance before it turns into diabetes, you may be able to get your cells to start heeding insulin's knock again by losing weight, exercising, and eating a well-rounded whole-foods diet—low in sugars, unhealthy fats, and refined carbohydrates, and rich in fruits and vegetables.

KEYS TO NATURAL BLOOD SUGAR CONTROL

In Chapter 2, you learned about the basics of a truly healthful diet. Those basics apply to people with diabetes or prediabetes as well. The rule of thumb: the more weight you want to lose and the more you are concerned about your health, the more you should cut refined carbs and sugars, and the more care you should take to eat low-glycemic foods. This is the step that makes the most difference for the most people, in my experience.

I put Gloria on a nearly zero-carbohydrate, no-grain "caveman" diet called the "Paleolithic" or "Paleo" diet. This diet was developed by Loren Cordain, Ph.D., who has written an excellent book on the subject called *The Paleo Diet* (Wiley, 2002). I added in the supplements I'll recommend later in this chapter. When she came to see me two months later, she looked thinner, especially around the middle. Her skin glowed and she moved with a spring in her step. She excitedly told me, "I have more energy than I've ever had!" My scale revealed that she had lost 15 pounds, and her own insulin had started to work better; her lab tests all came back within normal ranges.

Exercise is an important part of the puzzle for the insulin resistant *and* the diabetic. Even moderate exercise (such as brisk walking) enhances insulin sensitivity, as does resistance training with weights.

DRUGS FOR DIABETES AND THE NUTRIENTS THEY DEPLETE

If you have a diagnosis of diabetes or insulin resistance, also known as "prediabetes," borderline diabetes, metabolic syndrome, or Syndrome X, you should *not* head right for the pharmacy. It's been proven over and over that you can reverse this condition yourself, with the right diet, plus exercise. Speak to your doctor, and enroll him or her as your partner here.

Specific supplements, which you'll find in the last pages of this chapter, can help your body deal with insulin resistance. If, however, you are already taking an oral hypoglycemic, make sure you read this section carefully to see how to overcome any nutrient depletions. Whether you rely on medicines or not, sticking to a healthy diet and workout regimen are both crucial aspects of your treatment. They'll help you meet your daily quota of essential nutrients, and will help to prevent heart disease, nerve damage, and eye damage—all common complications with diabetes. The sooner you start eating right and exercising, the sooner you'll be feeling better, and possibly—with your doctor's help—reducing your medication dosages.

CLASSES OF DRUGS FOR BLOOD SUGAR CONTROL

In prescribing medication, most physicians will start with one class of drug and move down the line until they get the desired result. I'll give you the information you need on each drug, including how they're prescribed, side effects you might expect, and nutrients they deplete. Then, since most of these drugs deplete similar nutrients, I'll address those nutrients collectively at the end of the drug section.

ORAL ANTIDIABETIC DRUGS OR ORAL HYPOGLYCEMICS:
metformin (Glucophage, Glucophage XR, and Glucovance)

This drug is the most popular oral antidiabetic drug in America, with nearly 35 million prescriptions for the generic form alone in the year 2006. Like many drugs, it has a plant origin; it's derived from the French lilac plant, which has been used to treat diabetes since antiquity.

Actions: Metformin increases insulin sensitivity, encouraging cells to let sugars in when insulin is present; and it reduces the amount of glucose (simple sugars) absorbed into the body from food. Overall, it enhances the action of insulin and reduces blood sugar. It causes less weight gain and fewer episodes of hypoglycemia (low blood sugar) than any other medicine discussed in this chapter. It also has been found to protect against diabetic complications (neuropathy, retinopathy, kidney damage), and to lengthen lifespan in overweight people with type 2 diabetes.

Side effects: Gastrointestinal side effects are common with metformin.

A high percentage of those who take it experience nausea, vomiting, and diarrhea. To reduce the likelihood of these unpleasant side effects, start with low doses and gradually work up to higher doses.

Nutrients depleted: Metformin depletes vitamin B_{12} and folate, also known as folic acid. It reduces a substance called *intrinsic factor* in the stomach, which is needed for good absorption of B_{12} by the small intestine. A study published in the *Archives of Internal Medicine* in 2006 showed that diabetics on metformin had average B_{12} levels that were less than half of those of people who weren't taking any medication. The longer the drug had been used and the higher the dose, the greater the drop in B_{12}. Metformin may also deplete the body of the antioxidant and cardiovascular protector coenzyme Q_{10} (CoQ_{10}).

Supplements needed: Take vitamin B_{12} (200–1,000 micrograms [mcg]), folic acid (400–800 mcg), and CoQ_{10} (30–200 milligrams [mg]).

SULFONYLUREAS: chlorpropamide (Diabinese), glimepiride (Amaryl), glipizide (Glucotrol), and glyburide (DiaBeta, Micronase, or Glynase)

These drugs may be used as first-line therapies in patients who are not overweight, or as a second-line therapy—either instead of or in addition to metformin—in those who fail to get adequate blood sugar control with metformin. Sulfonylureas work best in patients who are not very insulin resistant. However, it isn't often used on its own.

Actions: Sulfonylureas stimulate the insulin-producing cells of the pancreas to release more insulin. They may also keep insulin in the bloodstream for a longer time, reduce insulin's release of fats (such as triglycerides and LDL) into the bloodstream, and reduce production of sugars in the liver. Other medications that work by this same mechanism include repaglinide (Prandin) and nateglinide (Starlix).

Side effects: Long-acting drugs in this group may cause low blood sugar—their effect on blood sugars may be too powerful for some patients. On the other hand, shorter-acting versions may not adequately lower blood sugar. These medicines can cause water weight gain (edema), gastrointestinal problems, and headaches.

Nutrient depleted: Sulfonylureas are suspected of depleting the body of the antioxidant and cardiovascular protector CoQ_{10}.

Supplements needed: Take CoQ_{10} (30–200 mg).

THIAZOLIDINEDIONES: pioglitazone (Actos), pioglitazone and glimepride (Duetact), rosiglitazone (Avandia), rosiglitazone and glimepiride (Avandaryl), and rosiglitazone and metformin (Avandamet)

This is another class of drugs used to control blood sugar. They are usually second- or third-line treatments, used in combination with metformin or sulfonylureas—or with both.

Actions: Thiazolidinediones can be described as insulin sensitizers—medications that promote better insulin sensitivity. They also reduce blood pressure and help to reduce inflammation within the blood vessels, both key factors in the progression of heart disease.

Side effects: Thiazolidinediones have been the subject of a great deal of controversy in recent years. There is now an FDA mandatory "black box" warning on this entire class of drugs regarding their serious cardiac effects. In 2007, a study was released that found that Avandia appears to increase risk of heart failure, heart attack, and death from heart attack. If these results are correct, as many as 60,000 to 100,000 heart attacks could be blamed on the effect of this drug.

Another drug in this class, Rezulin (troglitazone), was found to cause liver damage and liver failure, and was withdrawn.

Besides their potential to cause damage to the heart and liver, other side effects include weight gain—sometimes, extreme weight gain—a common issue with any hypoglycemic drug; water retention (edema) that causes swelling and can contribute to heart failure; sizeable increase in "bad" LDL cholesterol (about 19 percent more than placebo), bad news for heart health; and a slight decrease in levels of *hemoglobin*, a protein that transports oxygen through the bloodstream—another factor that could cause stress to the heart.

A decision to use any medication is about balancing risks with benefits. Increased awareness of heart risks with this class of drugs may help physicians to more closely monitor diabetics for problems, and to catch them before they're life threatening.

Nutrients depleted: None reported.

ALPHA-GLUCOSE INHIBITORS: acarbose (Precose), miglitol (Glyset)

Alpha-glucose inhibitors are prescribed alone or in combination with the other medications described in this chapter.

Actions: These drugs slow or block the breakdown of starches and some sugars. Taking them with the first bite of a meal slows the rise in blood sugars after eating, making the glucose curve rise and fall less steeply.

Side effects: Reactions include gas, bloating, abdominal pain, and diarrhea. These effects are usually worse when first starting to take the medicine, dissipating over time. A benefit of drugs in this class is that they don't cause blood sugars to dip too low on their own—but hypoglycemia can be a problem when it's coupled with other medicines for type 2 diabetes.

Nutrients depleted: None reported.

HORMONE: insulin (Lantus, Humalog, Novolog, Lispro-PFC, Levemir, Apidra, and other variations on these)

When oral diabetes medications don't control blood sugars adequately, injectable insulin might become a necessary part of your life. It might be added to one or more oral medications, or may be used alone.

Why don't doctors start type 2 diabetics on insulin in the first place— if oral antidiabetic drugs carry so many risks and can end up failing to control blood sugars adequately? First of all, because type 2 diabetics are already making insulin; the issue is being able to use it properly. In addition, controlling blood sugars with insulin is a tricky business. Just ask any insulin-dependent type 1 diabetic, who may have been injecting him or herself with insulin several times a day since childhood. A little too much insulin can throw you into dangerous low blood sugar, and if you don't get some glucose into your body quickly, you could fall into a coma and die. Use of insulin requires more strict self-monitoring and medical care, and is a treatment of last resort. Given insulin's risks, your medical team will try to make the most of the insulin your body can make, and will try to increase your cells' sensitivity to it, before prescribing it.

Even if you require insulin therapy, *don't give up on weight loss, a healthful diet, supplements, and exercise.* These measures are every bit as important to your health as they are to the person who is prediabetic, and you are much less likely to develop the devastating complications of diabetes. Don't believe for a minute that "it's OK to cheat, I'll just increase my insulin." Any responsible doctor will tell you that you'll be digging your own grave, one cookie at a time.

Actions: Injected insulin mimics that made by the body, allowing glucose to pass from the blood where there is too much glucose and into cells.

Side effects: Hypoglycemia, where blood sugars drop too low, making you shaky, lightheaded, and sweaty. Low blood sugar also causes rapid heartbeat, headache, and slurred speech, and can lead to coma and even, death. This side effect is treated with glucose tablets, which quickly get the blood sugar back up to normal.

Nutrients depleted: None reported.

WHY DO WE NEED B VITAMINS?

Even before you took these medications, you may have been deficient in several of these vitamins. Here's a primer on the most important B vitamins, including what they do in the body, and how to restore appropriate levels of each.

Vitamin B_{12} (Cyanocobalamin)

The B_{12} molecule is the largest and most complex of all of the vitamin molecules. Sources in the human diet include seafood, poultry, and dairy products. Little or none is found in plant foods.

You don't need much of this nutrient, and your body is capable of storing it. Deficiency can take a long time to occur in a generally healthy young person. But when you combine the B_{12}-reducing effects of metformin with the common reduction in B_{12} absorption that happens with aging, you're at risk.

Even in aging people who do not use metformin, there is a risk of deficiency due to poor absorption of nutrients, particularly vitamin B_{12}. It's estimated that 10 to 15 percent of people over sixty are deficient in B_{12}. In fact, many older people who think they're having "senior moments" could restore at least some of their mental sharpness with a B_{12} supplement.

Vitamin B_{12} is important for cancer prevention, as it enhances the stability of DNA, the genetic material found in each cell. DNA changes are where cancer starts. Vitamin B_{12} is also essential for proper nervous system function; it helps to build the *myelin sheath*, the fatty, conductive coating that enables nerve cells to send information efficiently. Symptoms of severe B_{12} deficiency include memory loss, numbness or tingling of the arms or legs, difficulty walking, mood swings, and dementia. Lack of this nutrient is one cause of anemia. It may contribute to *neuropathy*, a common and potentially painful consequence of diabetes. Serious deficiency can also cause constipation, sore tongue, and loss of appetite, probably due to changes in the GI tract lining.

Anyone with B_{12} levels below 150 picomoles per liter (pmol/L) is considered deficient. But you don't need to test your levels, especially if you are using metformin or have diabetes: chances are very good that adding more will improve your health. Your doctor should also look at the size of the red cell on a complete blood count (CBC). Extra large red cells are a sign of "macrocytic" or "large cell" anemia. That is, the B_{12}-deficient red cells enlarge in order to carry more oxygen. Their bigger size make them less flexible, and unable to reach the ends of the smaller capillaries. The result? Less oxygen to many of the cells of the body, including those oxygen-hungry heart and brain cells.

The RDA for vitamin B_{12} is 2.4 mcg a day, so you can get enough into the body with a dose of 200 to 500 mcg a day. You can use 1,000 mcg or more per day without fear of harm. There is no evidence of toxicity with this vitamin, although there may be some potential for imbalance between B_{12} and the other B vitamins. Always accompany a B_{12} supplement with a B-complex-containing multivitamin.

As you restore your B_{12}, inform your doctor, since changes in levels of this nutrient can lead to hypoglycemia. This is best measured by a blood test that looks at *glycosylated hemoglobin,* or HbA1C. This reflects levels of blood sugar over four weeks or so, rather than simply at the moment of the blood test.

Folic Acid/Folate

Although the terms are used interchangeably, strictly speaking, folic acid is the form found in supplements, while folate is found in foods. Most evidence suggests that folic acid is more bioavailable than folate, so with folic acid from supplements, you get more bang for your nutritional buck.

It's well known that five or more servings per day of fruits and vegetables is a known cancer-risk reducer, and this is likely due in part to the fact that these foods are excellent sources of folate. Leafy greens are the best source of all—the name "folate" actually is derived from the word "foliage." Beans, citrus juices, and whole grains are also good sources.

Like vitamin B$_{12}$, folate is a key player in the synthesis of DNA and in methylation (a biological process that helps DNA resist cancerous changes)—therefore, it's important for cancer prevention. Low folic acid levels in the body are linked with cancers of the cervix, colon, rectum, esophagus, lung, brain, breast, and pancreas.

Folic acid helps to prevent heart disease, too. A study of nearly 2,000 Finnish men found that those who got the most folate in their diets had about 45 percent as much risk of a heart attack, compared with men who ate the least folate. Studies have shown that high folate intake reduces risk of high blood pressure.

Folate adequacy is believed to help prevent memory loss and impaired thinking as we age. A study of the brains of thirty nuns who had had Alzheimer's disease found a strong association between the amount of atrophy (wasting) in the brain and folate levels in those tissues.

According to nutrition surveys of thousands of Americans, we aren't getting enough folate in our diets. On average, adults in the United States consume just under 300 mcg per day, and the RDA—the bare minimum intake—is 400 mcg per day. Folate intake has improved a good deal since wheat flour and cereals began to be fortified with this nutrient; but if you're diabetic, you should reduce your consumption of these simpler carbs. As you do so, make sure to add folate in the form of leafy greens, other vegetables, fruit, and a nutritional supplement.

Vitamin B$_6$ (Pyridoxine)

This nutrient, like the other B vitamins, plays multiple roles in the human body, supporting about 100 different enzymatic reactions and helping to make both mood-boosting (serotonin, dopamine, norepinephrine) and calming (gamma-aminobutyric acid, or GABA) neurotransmitters.

Vitamin B$_6$ is also needed to "burn" proteins for energy; for the transport of oxygen around the body; and for the building of another B vitamin, niacin. Vitamin B$_6$ is also needed to make DNA and for the proper function of the hormones estrogen and testosterone. Low B$_6$ is associated with poor immune function.

Outright deficiency is rare, since vitamin B$_6$ is found in a wide variety of foods, including bananas, fish, chicken, potatoes, spinach, and nuts. Taking 10 to 25 mg per day with your folate and B$_{12}$ should be enough. (Vitamin B$_6$ alone will not reduce levels of the heart-harmful amino acid homocysteine; more on this below.) There is substantial evidence that higher-dose B_6 could be helpful for treatment of diabetic nerve damage (neuropathy); vitamin B_6 inhibits the formation of glycosylated proteins, which damage nerves in diabetes. B_6 may help to prevent diabetic eye damage. It is also effective for premenstrual syndrome (PMS) and pregnancy-induced morning sickness; other research shows that higher-dose B_6 could be helpful for people who are depressed or who have carpal tunnel syndrome.

You and your doctor may agree to try a higher dose of B_6 if there's the potential for benefit. Up to 100 mg per day is safe, but should be combined with the other B vitamins as well for balance.

The B Vitamin-Homocysteine Connection

A common amino acid called methionine is converted in the body to a dangerous chemical called *homocysteine*. When levels of vitamins B_{12}, folate, and B_6 are adequate in the body, homocysteine is quickly converted into non-toxic amino acids. When these vitamins are depleted, homocysteine levels rise, and over time this contributes to serious problems such as heart disease, stroke, hypertension, and Alzheimer's disease. People who take metformin may be at increased risk of high homocysteine because of B_{12} and folate depletion.

A persistent rise in homocysteine levels of about 3 micromoles per liter (mmol/L) is believed to raise risk of heart attack about 10 percent, and to raise risk of stroke risk by 20 percent, in people who are not diabetic. One study found that for every 10 percent increase in homocysteine levels, there was a similar increase in risk of heart disease. The risks from excess homocysteine are even greater in people with diabetes.

Homocysteine is directly harmful to blood vessel walls. To find out how this amino acid affects the interior of arteries, refer to page 72 in Chapter 4, which deals with medications for heart attack prevention.

High homocysteine levels also seem to contribute to *neuropathy*, the nerve damage that can cause pain, numbness, or blindness in diabetes patients; and with *deep vein thrombosis* (a clot getting lodged in a vein); and *pulmonary embolism* (when a clot gets stuck in a blood vessel in the lungs).

Vitamin B_{12} and folate work together to keep homocysteine within healthy limits. A review of twelve studies where B vitamins were used to lower homocysteine found that taking 500 to 5,000 mcg of folate per day had the strongest effect, and that adding another 500 mcg of B_{12} to the mix lowered levels by an additional 7 percent. When you consider how big a difference even a small change in homocysteine can make in terms of heart attack and stroke risk, these doses of nutrients translate to big protection.

Diabetics are already likely to have high homocysteine, especially when they also have high blood pressure or cardiovascular disease. Metformin, with its B_6- and B_{12}-depleting effects, may add even more to the big picture of heart attack, stroke, or blood clots in diabetics. Metformin users are warned in the package information of their medicine that they have increased risk of death from these causes, compared to diabetics who are treated with diet alone or with diet plus insulin injections.

Good news: you can restore your B_6, B_{12}, and folic acid levels easily. This will reduce homocysteine and your risk of heart attacks and strokes, as well as helping to get your blood pressure within healthy limits. Following are the B vitamin doses for homocyteine lowering.

Dose: Folic acid (400 mcg), vitamin B_{12} (200–1,000 mcg), vitamin B_6 (10–25 mg).

OTHER SUPPLEMENTS FOR BETTER BLOOD-SUGAR CONTROL

People with diabetes can benefit from the comprehensive support a multivitamin. Diabetics are less able to fight off infections than non-diabetics. It seems that a multivitamin can boost diabetics' immunity and resistance to infection. In one revealing study, only 17 percent of diabetics who took multivitamins reported having an infection—such as a cold, the flu, or a stomach flu—while 93 percent who took a placebo (dummy) pill *did* report having one. This same study found that 89 percent of diabetics who took the dummy pill missed at least one day of work during the one-year study, while *none* of the multivitamin users missed work in that time period! This sounds like cheap and simple enough insurance! (To read more, see www.diabetesincontrol.com/modules.php?name=News&file=article&sid=10070.)

Following are other nutrients to benefit diabetics:

Vitamin B_1 (Thiamine)

The B vitamin thiamine is found in wheat germ, yeast, rice, wheat and other whole grain cereals, nuts, peas, leafy vegetables, apples, and bananas. A study by British researchers found that both type 1 and type 2 diabetics had blood levels of thiamine that were 75 percent below normal. When thiamine was added to the food of diabetic lab animals, kidney damage (common in diabetics) was cut by 70 to 80 percent.

Thiamine and a fat-soluble form of this nutrient, *benfotiamine*, help prevent the many complications of diabetes due to problems in circulation: blindness, kidney failure, and gangrene (leading to amputations). Currently, 20,000 diabetics go blind each year because of diabetic retinopathy, and amputations are common in those with the disease. For greatest benefit, thiamine must be taken in supplement form and as benfotiamine, which is lipid (or fat) soluble—a form that is better at getting into the cells than the water-soluble form.

Dose: Take vitamin B_1 as benfotiamine, 320 mg daily in divided doses (meaning 160 mg, twice daily).

Chromium

This mineral is found in foods such as romaine lettuce, onions, tomatoes, Brewer's yeast, oysters, liver, whole grains, and bran cereals. Because food-processing methods remove the naturally occurring mineral, many Westerners have low levels of this mineral. Deficiency is especially common in diabetics; chromium lack can create insulin resistance and poor blood sugar balance.

Chromium supplements can improve blood sugar levels. Of fifteen studies, twelve found at least some positive effect of chromium supplementation on various aspects of diabetes. In my own clinical experience, I have found chromium to be very helpful in fighting sugar cravings.

Dose: Take 200 mcg per day.

Vanadium

This trace mineral is, like chromium, essential for insulin's actions on lowering blood sugar. It's found in a wide variety of foods, including seafood, meat, dairy, cooking oils, and fresh fruits and vegetables. It is often low in diabetics; in those cases, it should be supplemented.

Dose: Take 10 mg of vanadyl sulfate (most common form) daily, yielding 2 mg of vanadium.

Magnesium

The American Diabetes Association reports that 25 percent of diabetics are magnesium deficient (although other figures place this much higher), and that supplementing with this mineral can improve blood sugar control. Green vegetables such as spinach are good sources of magnesium, because the center of the chlorophyll molecule (which gives green vegetables their color) contains magnesium. Some legumes (beans and peas), nuts and seeds, and whole, unrefined grains are also good sources of magnesium.

Dose: Take 500–600 mg daily; the most common form found in supplements is magnesium oxide (that's what milk of magnesia is made from). It may give you loose stools; if so, switch to a form such as magnesium glycinate or citrate which is bound or chelated (pronounced *kee-lated*) to an amino acid.

Coenzyme Q_{10}

This nutrient is made in every body cell; it also is depleted by sulfonylurea drugs and metformin. If you are taking these drugs or the statin drugs commonly prescribed to lower cholesterol (which also deplete CoQ_{10}), read a detailed description in the section Coenzyme Q_{10}: Don't Take Your Statin without It! on page 66, in Chapter 4. Diabetics will generally benefit from this nutrient, as it strengthens the heart and helps both to lower blood pressure and increase energy levels. CoQ_{10} is not found in any significant quantity in food.

Dose: Take 30–200 mg per day.

Alpha-lipoic acid (ALA)

Diabetics are under greater oxidative stress than non-diabetics; in other words, their cells crank out more free radicals. The damage these free radicals do helps to explain many diabetic complications. Diabetics require strong antioxidant protection, and alpha-lipoic acid fits this bill. This "super antioxidant" has been found to have healing effects on neuropathy in diabetics, as well as to control insulin resistance. Food sources include spinach, broccoli, beef, yeast (particularly Brewer's yeast), and certain organ meats (such as the kidney and heart). It is made in small amounts in the body. ALA works together with vitamins E and C, enhancing the body's overall ability to neutralize free radicals. ALA has also been found to help insulin work better, and to promote production of glutathione, a powerful antioxidant made in the liver. *Its use even in medication-dependent diabetics has been shown to reduce complications.*

Caution: Please let your doctor know that you're taking ALA, and monitor blood sugar levels carefully, since it can lower your need for insulin or other diabetic medications. I've seen this occur in my own patients, and it can be a cause for alarm if you aren't prepared. Even though you obviously want your blood sugar lowered, you also don't want it to be pushed unexpectedly low by this combination. You and your doctor can work out a lower dose of medication, be it oral or insulin, as you gradually start using the ALA. It has no side effects. I would *strongly* recommend it to every diabetic.

Dose: Take 200–600 mg per day.

Other Antioxidants

A broad spectrum of antioxidants—vitamins C, E, mixed carotenes (found in colorful vegetables and fruit), proanthocyanidins (found in grape seed extract), curcumin (from the herb turmeric), and catechins (found in tea, particularly the green variety)—is useful to round out any diabetic's supplement program. The various antioxidants work together, like instruments in an orchestra; taking one or two isn't enough. For best results, take a combination of antioxidants. You can take a whole-food antioxidant supplement. a green drink powder, for example, or a supplement that contains a variety of food-based antioxidants for maximum benefit.

THE DIABETES SUPPLEMENT PROGRAM

Diabetics can benefit from a high-potency multivitamin as described in Chapter 2 (supplemented with high enough doses of B vitamins to lower homocysteine), plus a few other specific supplements (discussed above) to match the doses of the following nutrients. In many cases, prediabetic patients have resolved their problems with this natural approach (including diet changes and exercise as described earlier in this chapter) and no longer need drugs.

I was taken aback recently while reading an interview of a forty-four-year-old diabetic wife and mother who was on oral hypoglyemics. Her photograph showed her on a bicycle (great!) but still obviously overweight. She was quoted as admitting, "I've not been able to eliminate sugar. For me, it's like a drug." How sad! Like many diabetics, she figures that diet is less important, as long as she's taking her medication. My suggestion? If she were to take the appropriate supplements, I'd almost guarantee that her sugar cravings would disappear. She'd be able to lose weight, and perhaps get off the medication for good.

Take daily in divided doses, best with breakfast and dinner, one-half dose each time:

- Alpha-lipoic acid: 200–600 mg

- Chromium: 200 mcg

- Coenzyme Q_{10}: 30–200 mg

- Folic acid: 400 mcg

- Magnesium: 500–600 mg

- Mixed antioxidant supplement

- Vitamin B_1: 320 mg (as benfotiamine)

- Vitamin B_6: 10–25 mg

- Vitamin B_{12}: 200 mcg

- Vanadium: 2 mg

Anyone with diabetes needs to take extra-good care of his or her heart. The chapter following this one deals with this topic in detail, describing the ways in which high cholesterol, high blood pressure, and inflammation can threaten your heart's health—and how controlling these factors with diet and supplements can do a great deal to protect your heart for many years to come. I strongly recommend that you read the next chapter as well as this one.

Beyond just "handling" your type 2 diabetes—essentially, a disease of civilization—you now see how it can be controlled, if not totally eliminated, by correct diet, supplements, and lifestyle. If you need to use medications to help, you should also follow a diet and supplement program designed to replenish drug-induced and disease-induced depletions. This will go a long way toward increasing the quality of your life.

FOUR

Prescriptions for Cardiovascular Health: Drugs for High Cholesterol and Hypertension

At a recent business luncheon, I ended up seated next to Mark, a slightly overweight, greying, fifty-six-year-old accountant. He proudly ordered everything "low-fat and non-fat, oil on the side," along with a diet soda, and expounded to me at some length about his doctor's advice regarding weight loss and heart disease prevention. He told me that his medication, Lipitor, had lowered his total cholesterol to under 200. "My dad died young from heart disease," he told me, "and I sure am glad I know what to do to prevent the same thing from happening to me."

I did my best to listen politely. Mark wasn't my patient, after all, and he seemed so happy and secure with the advice his doctor had given him. I didn't want to rock his boat.

"Are you working out, too?" I asked him, noting to myself that he was not looking very fit or toned.

"That part's been harder," he replied. "Lately—and maybe it's just age—I've been having sore muscles, and it's not just after I work out, either. Plus, my energy isn't what it used to be."

That's when I realized that I had to speak up. I knew that his muscle pain and fatigue probably weren't just from getting older. "I hope you don't mind my saying so, but your sore muscles are most likely a side effect of the Lipitor."

"Why would Lipitor make my muscles hurt?"

"Because it interferes with the production of coenzyme Q_{10}."

I was met with a blank look. Predictably, he had no idea what coenzyme Q_{10} (CoQ_{10}) was. I explained that it's a nutrient required by every cell of the body to transform carbohydrate and fat into energy, in the many "energy-producing factories" called *mitochondria;* and that the same mechanism Lipitor employs to lower cholesterol also lowers production of CoQ_{10}.

He was actually grateful for the information, and wondered why his doctor hadn't recommended that he take CoQ_{10} along with the drug. "I'm constantly amazed at how little attention most physicians pay to their patients' nutrient status," I told him, "and it's affected by the drugs they prescribe. For me, this is as least as important as the prescription itself."

I didn't stop there, either, seeing my opportunity to make a significant difference in this man's life, and he was asking for more information. "Now, about your diet," I explained. "The idea that eating high-cholesterol foods leads to elevated blood levels of cholesterol and causes heart disease may be common medical wisdom. But eating foods that contain cholesterol not only doesn't raise your cholesterol levels—it doesn't cause heart disease, either."

At this point Mark didn't know what to believe. "Are you saying that I can eat eggs and butter, with no risk to my heart?" He looked amazed. And I could already see him casting an eager eye on the bread and butter at the center of the table. I realized that I'd better be more precise.

"Hold on . . . I can see you ogling that bread basket!"

He was caught! Laughing, he replied, "Okay—no bread. Tell me why, Doc."

"Although you don't have to worry too much about the butter, you shouldn't touch that bread with a ten-foot pole!" I told him that his current 'low-fat insurance policy' was in fact, not very useful as a protection against heart attacks and stroke, nor was cutting fat out of his diet. "If you look at recent research, the cause of heart disease isn't cholesterol: it's *inflammation,* caused by *excess intake of sugar and other simple carbs,* like those crusty white dinner rolls. The inflammation leads to insulin resistance, weight gain, diabetes, and heart disease."

I sure rocked his boat—and he thanked me for it. I let him know where to check out the research (listed here) that he could then take to his doctor to discuss a different approach to his condition.

By the way, I often don't get thanked for such interventions, so I especially appreciated Mark's openness and enthusiasm. The usual responses can be anything from, "My doctor is the best and who are you to tell me differently?" to "You're telling me I have to make even more changes? Forget it!" Or "That's not what I've read, so you must be wrong." He went on to make better choices for himself and seeing the results, became a believer. When I ran into him a few months later, he'd lost his beer belly, gained some muscle, and was pain free.

DOES DIETARY CHOLESTEROL CAUSE HEART DISEASE?

It can take years, even decades, for the medical status quo to catch up with the cutting edge of medical and nutritional research. Just ask any medical pioneer whose radical ideas were ridiculed . . . until everyone else finally started to see the light.

The enormous use of statin drugs in the United States is tied into the belief that lowering cholesterol by any means necessary will, for virtually every person, dramatically reduce the chances of having a stroke or heart attack. But the cutting edge of research, which I'm sure will become accepted as fact in not too long, shows that the link between cholesterol and heart disease has been greatly exaggerated.

High cholesterol counts are indicative of increased heart disease risk, but it appears that we've been looking at the equation backwards: *high blood fats are an effect, not a cause, of elevated cardiovascular risk.* And the evidence strongly suggests that high cholesterol is a result of excess inflammation in the body. That excess inflammation seems to be a more likely root cause of dangerous changes in the cardiovascular system.

You don't have to go any further than the medical literature—the dozens of studies published each month in medical journals and presented at medical conferences—to see this. It just hasn't hit the mainstream's radar yet. You now have the inside scoop: when you're concerned about preventing heart disease, think *reduce inflammation,* not *lower cholesterol.*

If you chose to read this chapter, you are probably one of the millions of American adults who take a statin and/or a blood pressure-lowering drug every day. You've probably made this choice based on your doctor telling you that not lowering your cholesterol and/or blood pressure will eventually lead you down the road to heart attack or stroke. Perhaps you've made a shift to a low-fat diet based on that doctor's advice, rejecting eggs, whole-milk dairy products, butter, and meat in favor of "reduced-cholesterol egg products," skim milk, margarine, and foods made mostly with processed grains. Here's what your doctor may not have told you:

- A review of five big studies found that the risk of non-fatal heart attack and stroke was reduced by 1.4 percent in people on statin therapy—but that the rate of serious adverse effects *rose* 1.8 percent in those same people. (Serious adverse effect: any medication side effect that results in death, is life threatening, requires hospitalization, or results in persistent or significant health problems.) Not a great trade-off.

- There is no relationship between blood cholesterol and heart disease risk in women over fifty or in men over seventy. Statins given to these individuals are not only wasted, but expose them to risk of side effects that isn't outweighed by benefit to their hearts.

- A survey of South Carolina adults found no correlation of blood cholesterol levels with "bad" dietary habits, such as use of red meat, animal fats, fried foods, butter, eggs, whole milk, bacon, sausage, and cheese. Does that sound like heresy, or what?

- A Medical Research Council survey showed that men eating butter ran half the risk of developing heart disease compared with those using margarine.

- Mother's milk provides a higher proportion of cholesterol than almost any other food. It also contains over 50 percent of its calories as fat, much of it saturated fat. Both cholesterol and saturated fat are essential for growth in babies and children, especially for the development of the brain. Yet, the American Heart Association is now recommending that children consume a low-cholesterol, low-fat diet—exactly the kind of diet that was linked, in one recent study, with failure to thrive in children. The fact is, children need good fats to provide the raw materials for healthy brain cells.

Statins *have* been found to help with heart attack and stroke prevention in two groups of people: those with type 2 diabetes, and those who have already had a heart attack or stroke and want to prevent another one. The catch is that the drugs probably don't help these people because they lower cholesterol, but because they address another, more important risk factor: inflammation.

However, even this action is open to question. The statins may be changing the results of commonly used tests for measuring inflammation (C-reactive protein tests, for example; more on this below), rather than actually altering the inflammation itself. In other words, we've lowered the marker, but the underlying inflammatory condition remains.

THE INFLAMMATION CONNECTION

Inflammation is the immune system's response to injury. It sends a repair crew to the point of injury, breaks down injured and dead tissue, kills bacteria, and makes way for the healing response. This process can happen anywhere in the body, and it has a great impact on the health of the blood vessels that feed the heart muscle—the vessels that cause heart attack when blocked by plaques, which are scab-like thickened areas that grow inside the walls of arteries.

When I spot someone with obvious signs of metabolic syndrome—usually a middle-aged person with a big stomach—I know that a lot of inflammation is going on in the person's body, and that he or she is at high risk of heart disease and high blood pressure. Mark fell into this category; so do "apple-shaped" women who carry their fat in their bellies, such as Gloria in the last chapter. (The more typical "pear" shape, where fat is stored in the legs and buttocks, seems to protect against heart problems in women.)

Fat cells in the belly, also called *visceral* fat, create a lot of inflammation. If you're insulin resistant or diabetic, the state of high insulin and high blood sugar is creating even worse inflammation. This inflammation creates plaques in the twists and turns of the blood vessels that feed the muscular walls of the heart. This, in turn, drastically increases your risk of having a heart attack.

Where does that "bad" LDL (low-density lipoprotein) cholesterol come in? It's used as a sort of spackling and filling material within those plaques. Once there, it can contribute to the inflammatory process even more—especially if it has been attacked by free radicals (oxidized). The inflammatory process creates even more oxidation, a process similar to the rusting of iron, which in turn creates more damage and more inflammation. Keep in mind that high levels of LDL, triglycerides, and other bad fats in the blood are likely to be *effects* of the inflammation that is the real direct cause of heart disease.

We can determine how much inflammation is going on in your body using a simple lab test that measures levels of C-reactive protein (CRP). CRP is regarded as an important risk factor for heart disease, and a test for its levels in the blood is likely to soon be a standard part of any evaluation for cardiovascular disease.

Diet and Inflammation

The standard American diet is a pro-inflammatory diet. I'm not referring only to diets high in fat—although the usual high trans-fat, fast-food, and processed-food diet consumed in the United States is, in fact, pro-inflammatory. I'm also referring to the low-fat, high-carbohydrate, high-vegetable-oil diet that has been pushed on people at risk for heart disease—like Mark—for so many decades now.

The traditional high-fat diets consumed by Eskimos—almost entirely seal meat and fish—is heart healthy and anti-inflammatory. Seal meat and fish are loaded with beneficial omega-3 fatty acids. The Masai in Africa, who subsist on milk and meat, have healthy hearts and don't suffer from excess inflammation.

The fats you eat are directly transformed into chemicals in your body. Some of those chemicals promote inflammation; others calm it. Most nut, seed, and vegetable oils—the oils used to make processed foods—are rich in omega-6 polyunsaturated fats, which are almost always made into the chemicals that promote inflammation. Eating refined flour and sugar pushes more of the omega-6 fats you eat into the making of those inflammatory chemicals. This is one reason why refined flour and sugar are so bad for your health in so many ways. Also, if you're eating lots of margarine and food fried in corn oil, you're increasing the inflammation in your body. Modern diets tend to be quite high in the omega-6 fats and very low in omega-3s. (Olive and macadamia nut oils contain mostly omega-9 fatty acids that don't affect inflammation at all.)

Real, unprocessed, wild-caught or grass-grazed food from nature, fatty or not, is good for your heart. Factory-farmed cattle eat grain, which causes the fats in their meat and milk to accumulate more inflammatory omega-6 fats. In the days when milk and meat came from pasture-raised cattle, that milk and meat were full of those wonderful omega-3s, which are made into *anti-inflammatory* chemicals in the body. Omega-3 oils are found most plentifully in fish, flaxseeds, and walnuts; vegetables and algae also contain some omega-3s.

Think of omega-6 fats, sugars, and refined grains as slow-burning fires and omega-3 fats as cool, fresh, quenching water. And now imagine the standard American diet, which generally contains a ratio of omega-6 fats to omega-3 fats of about 20:1. This is a conflagration waiting to happen—if it isn't happening already. The drastic shift in fat and refined carbohydrate consumption over the last one hundred years brings the body to a slow-burning state of inflammation. As a result, any inflammation in the blood vessels is made worse.

A more appropriate balance of omega-6s to omega-3s is 2:1 to 3:1—a balance fulfilled by the diets consumed by our ancestors for most of history. That's the diet our bodies evolved on, and a diet that's worth trying to achieve for heart disease prevention today.

Food sensitivities can also cause an inflammatory response, so eliminating the common allergens, wheat and dairy products, is very helpful in reducing this inflammation. Both inflammation and the food sensitivities that can cause it may play a role in arthritis, as well; more on this in Chapter 5. To find out how to identify and eliminate foods to which you have sensitivities or allergies, turn to the section on the Elimination Diet, on page 97 in Chapter 6.

DRUGS FOR HEART DISEASE RISK FACTORS AND THE NUTRIENTS THEY DEPLETE

All this having been said, you may, in the short or long term, benefit from statins if:

1. You are diabetic.

2. You have had a heart attack.

3. You've been diagnosed with heart disease but have not had a heart attack.

If your blood pressure is high or borderline, keeping it down with drugs may be necessary as well. High blood pressure is dangerous and does damage to artery walls.

Both types of drugs deplete nutrients, which must be replenished, as you'll see next. Keep in mind, however, that you can also reduce your cholesterol and blood pressure with an appropriate diet and anti-inflammatory supplement program. Use the medicines if you must, but stick with the diet and supplement program I recommend . . . and *inform your physician that you are adding supplements. Then, he or she can monitor you more closely, to see if your medication needs to be decreased.*

CLASSES OF CHOLESTEROL-LOWERING DRUGS

Statin drugs are the most prescribed medicines for lowering cholesterol. In fact, Lipitor (generic name atorvastatin) is the top-selling drug *on the planet,* a $20 billion industry. They've been heralded as "miracle drugs" that reduce cholesterol counts and battle inflammation. Less frequently used drugs for high cholesterol include the bile acid sequestrants and fibrates.

BILE ACID SEQUESTRANTS: cholestyramine (Questran), colesevelan (Welchol), and colestipol (Colestid)

Bile acid sequestrants are sometimes used in combination with statins, and may be used alone in women who are pregnant or breastfeeding.

Actions: Bile acid sequestrants work by preventing cholesterol from being absorbed, and increasing the amount that's flushed out of the body.

Side effects: Common side effects include constipation and increased risk of dangerous bleeding (these drugs deplete vitamin K, which is needed for blood clotting); any pregnant or breastfeeding woman using bile acid sequestrants needs to be careful to replace depleted vitamins.

Nutrients depleted: These medications deplete the body of vitamins A, E, D, K, folic acid, calcium, iron, magnesium, vitamin B_{12}, and zinc. Other reports suggest reductions in omega-3 fatty acids and a 30 percent reduction in body levels of *carotenoids*, a class of antioxidant nutrients that includes beta-carotene.

Needed supplements: Take vitamin A (20,000 IU), vitamin E (100 milligrams [mg] in tocotrienol form, see below for more information), vitamin D (400–2,000 IU), folic acid (400 micrograms [mcg]), vitamin K (80 mcg), calcium (1,000 mg), iron (15 mg, if you're premenopausal), magnesium (400–600 mg), vitamin B_{12} (200 mcg), and zinc (25 mg), and omega-3 fatty acids (1,000–3,000 mg).

FIBRATES: bezafibrate (Bezalip), ciprofibrate (Modalim), clofibrate (Atromid-S), fenofibrate (TriCor), and gemfibrozil (Lopid)

These drugs work well to lower triglycerides and "bad" LDL and raise "good" HDL (high-density lipoproteins); they may be used with statins in diabetics because fibrates help to reduce insulin resistance.

Actions: These drugs work through a mechanism similar to those of some blood sugar-lowering (hypoglycemic) drugs.

Side effects: Fibrates have potential for serious side effects when combined with statins: they increase risk of *rhabdomyolysis*, a life-threatening breakdown of muscle tissue, and of *myopathy*, muscle pain and damage. As you'll see, both of these side effects are of concern with statins alone.

Nutrients depleted: Gemfibrozil depletes CoQ_{10} and vitamin E. Clofibrate has been found to deplete vitamin B_{12}.

Needed supplements: Take CoQ_{10} (100–300 mg), vitamin E (100 mg in tocotrienol form), and vitamin B_{12} (200 mcg).

STATINS: atorvastatin (Lipitor), fluvastatin (Lescol), lovastatin (Mevacor), pravastatin (Pravachol) rosuvastatin (Crestor), and simvastatin (Zocor)

At this writing, some 36 million Americans have cholesterol counts high enough to make them candidates for statin therapy. The guidelines for safe cholesterol levels continue to change so that more and more people are prescribed these medicines at higher and higher doses.

Actions: These drugs work reduce "bad" LDL and raise "good" HDL.

Side effects: Side effects include headache, rash, nausea, heartburn, constipation, diarrhea, gas, urinary tract infection, joint and muscle pain; changes in mood and thinking ability. For details on this last side effect, see the inset "Statins' Potential Effects on Mood and Thinking Ability" on page 66.

Nutrient depleted: Statins deplete the body of CoQ_{10}, causing some of their more worrisome side effects. The consequences of that deficiency are broad. It can translate to:

Heart failure. Deficiency of CoQ_{10} makes the heart less able to do its job, leading to congestive heart failure (CHF). CHF happens when the heart becomes too weak to efficiently pump blood through the whole cardiovascular system. Blood backs up and fluid accumulates in the lungs and throughout the body. In 1968, about 10,000 people died from CHF; in 1993, that figure increased to 42,000. Could CoQ_{10} depletion from statin therapy have played a role in this dramatic increase? The logic seems too compelling to dismiss.

In fact, CoQ_{10} is regarded as a valuable natural therapy for people with heart failure. Studies have shown increased risk of heart failure in statin users, and this is likely related to the CoQ_{10}-depleting effect of the drugs. It's essential to add the nutrient back in to help avoid this serious weakening of the heart's pumping power.

Muscle pain and weakness. As I explained to Mark, any person on statins who experiences significant new muscle pain, weakness, or tenderness should let his or her doctor know, as it may be a sign of muscle damage. Continuing to take the drug in spite of muscle damage can lead to *rhabdomyolysis,* a potentially fatal condition. If you have myopathy, taking CoQ_{10} is essential whether or not you continue on the drug. Myopathy is an obvious sign of CoQ_{10} depletion.

The good news is that CoQ_{10} is easy to supplement. In addition to protecting you against these side effects, this nutrient will improve your overall health as well. To learn more, see the following section on CoQ_{10}.

Needed supplement: Take 100–300 mg of CoQ_{10} daily.

COENZYME Q_{10}: DON'T TAKE YOUR STATIN WITHOUT IT!

Published scientific research leaves no doubt that statins lower CoQ_{10}.

Statins' Potential Effects on Mood and Thinking Ability

The side effects described below may or may not be related to CoQ_{10} depletion with statin drugs. Some experts believe that these effects on thinking and mood may have more to do with depletion of cholesterol, which is essential for brain cell function, or with the drug's effects on important body chemicals that influence our moods and thoughts.

Cognitive Problems

It's estimated that 15 percent of people who use statins have some reduction in their ability to think, reason, remember, and concentrate. It isn't unusual for doctors to tell these patients, "It isn't the medication—you're just getting older." But studies are now finding that this is a real side effect that can be reversed when the dose is lowered or the medicine is stopped.

Research from the University of Pittsburgh finds that people taking statins perform worse on tests of learning, cognition (thinking ability), and memory. One brilliant professor whose mental abilities went downhill after starting the drugs was sent to me for evaluation of his possible Alzheimer's disease. Instead, I took a careful drug history, saw the connection, and stopped his medication. I also added in some nutrients such as CoQ_{10}, fish oil, and other mind enhancers, as well as cholesterol-lowering nutrients. Luckily for him, he soon recovered his brain power, unlike others less fortunate.

The higher the dose, the greater the depletion, so the lowest effective statin dose is best.

The drugs lower cholesterol by inhibiting the action of the enzyme, called HMG-CoA, that is responsible for cholesterol production in the body. It just so happens that HMG-CoA is also needed to make CoQ_{10}. When you replenish CoQ_{10} with a supplement, you can diminish symptoms related to its lack.

What is CoQ_{10}, and what is its role in the body? It is a compound made within the cells of all animals. CoQ_{10} is fat-soluble, meaning that it is stored in fats. Cell membranes, which are mostly composed of fat, contain a great deal of CoQ_{10}, as do the lipids (fats) that travel around the body in the bloodstream—including both "good" (HDL) and "bad" (LDL) cholesterol.

A former NASA physician and astronaut, Duane "Doc" Graveline, had a similar experience and wrote *Statin Drugs: Side Effects and The Misguided War on Cholesterol* (Duane Graveline, 2006). We met at a recent medical conference, and I was impressed by his knowledge, sincerity, and dedication. He lectures around the country to warn others of this dangerous side effect of statins. A visit to his website, www.spacedoc.net, will give you lots more good information.

Irritability, Mood Swings, and Depression

Researchers at University of California at San Diego have collected a series of case studies of people who became very irritable while on statins. They became their normal selves again after discontinuing the drug, then became irritable again when the drug was reintroduced. These medicines can also change hormone balance in men in ways that cause them to grow female-like breasts.

Other problems that have been reported in statin users: peripheral neuropathy (numbness, pain, or tingling in extremities), sleep problems, sexual problems, fatigue, dizziness, unexplained swelling, shortness of breath, vision changes, weight change, changes in blood sugar or blood pressure, nausea, upset stomach, and ringing in the ears.

If you don't feel like yourself while on statins, don't let anyone tell you that it couldn't possibly be the effects of the medication. It could be, and it's worth consulting with your doctor about stopping the drug temporarily or at least lowering the dose to see whether it helps.

In short, CoQ_{10}:

- Is required for the transformation of carbohydrate and fat into energy at the cellular level; this happens in the many tiny *mitochondria* (energy-producing "factories"). There are hundreds of mitochondria in each heart muscle cell.

- Is also an antioxidant that is especially good at protecting cell membranes—which are made of fat—against free-radical damage.

- Has blood-thinning effects when taken as a supplement, which helps prevent heart attacks and some strokes.

- Works with vitamin E to prevent oxidation of fats throughout the body, providing improved protection against premature aging and chronic disease.

CoQ_{10} is found in many foods, mostly meats, vegetable oils (including soybean), fish, nuts, and some vegetables, but the daily intake of the average person through diet is below 5 mg—a fraction of the amount usually taken in supplement form (30 to 300 mg). It's estimated that only about 25 percent of the CoQ_{10} in your body is supplied through diet.

Supplements of CoQ_{10} restore normal levels of this nutrient in people who take statin drugs without reducing the drug's effect on cholesterol levels. Actually, research shows that the antioxidant, blood-thinning effect of CoQ_{10} in supplement form *plus* a statin reduce heart disease risk better than the drug alone. Starting both the CoQ_{10} supplement and the statin together can prevent depletion entirely.

Supplementing CoQ_{10} is easy and safe. It's non-toxic even at high doses. Possible, but uncommon, side effects may include mild inability to sleep, elevated liver enzyme levels, rashes, nausea, and upper abdominal pain.

Dose: If you take statins, take 100–300 mg per day of this nutrient. Use a version that's packaged with oil and vitamin E to ensure the best possible absorption, or use along with a multi that contains vitamin E. For best results, take your CoQ_{10} with a food containing fat, such as vegetables in butter, scrambled eggs, nuts, or nut butter.

NUTRIENTS TO LOWER CHOLESTEROL

By now, I hope you understand why the cholesterol-lowering issue is less important than addressing the underlying inflammation. Rather than targeting the symptom, we should address the underlying problem, in this case, inflammation. Don't shoot the messenger! If we treat the inflammation adequately, the cholesterol levels should normalize. If the HDL, the "good" cholesterol, is high, there's no problem. If LDL, the "bad" cholesterol, is high, antioxidants are key for preventing it from oxidizing or rusting and causing cell damage.

Here are some nutritional interventions to consider:

Omega-3 Fatty Acids

Studies show that omega-3s from fish oil helps decrease the inflammation associated with cardiovascular disease. The American Heart Association began recommending it as a treatment option in 2003.

Fish oil also lowers triglycerides. It protects against heart failure, irregular heartbeat (arrhythmia), heart attack, and sudden death. Studies show that fish oil supplements can be as effective as statins—and without any side effects. Regular intake of fish oil has been shown to lower the risk of cardiac-related death.

One study has raised doubts about the safety of fish oil for people who have severe angina (heart pains) or heart failure. If you have one of these conditions, consult with your doctor about this research before trying fish oil.

Dose: Take 2,000 mg daily.

Niacin

Niacin or nicotinic acid, one of the water-soluble B vitamins, namely B_3, improves levels of cholesterol ("bad" LDL drops by 10 to 20 percent and "good" HDL rises by 15 to 35 percent) and triglycerides (lower by 20 to 50 percent) when given in doses well above the basic vitamin requirement.

Niacin helps change other risk factors for heart disease. Levels of a very heart-toxic blood fat, *apolipoprotein (a)*, were significantly reduced (20 percent) by niacin, but were not altered by the drug used in the study (gemfibrozil, a fibrate drug). *Fibrinogen*, another risk factor, was reduced by niacin, but was *increased* 6 to 9 percent by gemfibrozil. The authors concluded that 2,000 mg of Niaspan, a time-released form of niacin, had a better effect on fibrinogen levels than the statin.

Niacin comes in both immediate-release and timed-release forms. There are some side effects you should know about:

1. A common and troublesome side effect of niacin is flushing, which can be decreased by taking it during or after meals or by taking an aspirin thirty minutes prior. Or, use a form of niacin called *inositol hexanicotinate* (IHN), a non-flushing form of niacin that is effective in somewhat lower doses.

2. Niacin can cause high blood sugar—so *don't take niacin if you have diabetes.*

3. Gastrointestinal symptoms such as nausea, indigestion, gas, vomiting, and diarrhea, and the activation of peptic ulcers are potential side effects. Liver problems and gout have also been reported with niacin therapy.

4. The effect of high blood pressure medicines may also be increased while you are on niacin, so monitor blood pressure while adjusting to your new niacin regimen.

Dose: Start at 100 mg and gradually increase to an average daily dose of 1.5 to 3 grams (1,500–3,000 mg). Be sure to consult with your doctor and have him or her monitor your levels of cholesterol and liver enzymes if you wish to try this therapy.

Sterols

Plant sterols are extracts of certain plants that, when ingested, interfere with the absorption of cholesterol in the small intestine. Thus, dietary cholesterol never gets into the system. Two plant sterols are now available in a spreadable form, as a substitute for margarine. In one study, people on statins took sterol tablets; they had an extra 9 percent reduction in LDL cholesterol and a 6 percent decline in total cholesterol.

Dose: Take 1.6–2.4 grams daily, from supplements or sterol-enriched spreads.

Tocotrienols

Tocotrienols are a form of the antioxidant vitamin E. Naturally found in palm oil and available as a supplement, research suggests that tocotrienols are the most potent antioxidants in the vitamin E family. They also show promise for cancer prevention, especially for breast and skin cancer. Studies have found that they can bring down LDL cholesterol counts through the same mechanism as statins, and that they protect the heart.

Dose: Take 100 mg per day of tocotrienols. This dose is fine to take in addition to the tocopherol form of vitamin E that's usually found in multivitamins.

D-Ribose

While we're on the topic of heart health, I'd like to introduce one of my favorite supplements, D-ribose. It works by helping your heart cells to produce energy. Just think of it: your heart muscle is beating at least sixty times a minute, twenty-four hours a day, three hundred sixty-five days a year. It never rests! So it has to be supplied with a continuous and reliable source of fuel.

Energy is made in the hundreds of mitochondria that live in each heart cell: it burns the food we eat, and gives off energy in the form of ATP. One of the building blocks of ATP is a form of sugar called D-ribose. Although it is found in small amounts in red meat, most of it is made in the body. When there is insufficient blood flow or oxygen supply, we can't make enough D-ribose to generate energy. The solution is to take D-ribose as a supplement.

D-ribose can boost heart function in those with coronary artery disease, hypertension, and those on statins. It also is useful for treating fibromyalgia, where there are pains all over due to lack of oxygen in the muscles and surrounding tissue. Athletes, especially marathon runners, love it. Combine your D-ribose with L-carnitine (see page 131) and CoQ_{10} for a great boost in energy.

Caution: Since D-ribose can lower blood sugar, diabetics need to monitor their insulin levels when taking it.

Dose: Take 5 grams (approximately 1 teaspoon of powder) twice daily; it's best mixed with orange juice.

DRUGS FOR BLOOD PRESSURE CONTROL AND THE NUTRIENTS THEY DEPLETE

Hypertension, the medical term for high blood pressure, is a serious condition. Normal blood pressure is about 120/80. If your blood pressure is above 140 systolic (that's the top number) or 90 diastolic (the bot-

Homocysteine and Heart Disease Risk

If you read Chapter 3, you already know that high levels of an amino acid called *homocysteine* are linked to heart disease risk. A natural product of protein metabolism in the body, homocysteine can accumulate when there aren't enough B vitamins to break it down into harmless byproducts. Controlling homocysteine levels in the body is an important part of heart health.

Homocysteine affects the walls of arteries in at least four ways:

1. By doing direct damage to the cells that line the arteries, making them vulnerable to the formation of *plaque*, scab-like growths on the inner artery wall that can slow or stop blood flow to the heart.

2. By affecting the "tightness" and flexibility of blood vessels. High homocysteine appears to reduce the production of *nitric oxide*, a beneficial chemical that plays a role in reducing blood pressure and opening blood vessels wider to allow more blood to pass through.

3. By affecting the "stickiness" of blood. When levels of *clotting factors* rise, blood becomes stickier and thicker and clots become more likely. Clots can then become lodged in narrowed blood vessels, triggering a heart attack or stroke.

4. By increasing levels of free radicals in the body. Homocysteine is known to enhance the production of free radicals—the unpaired electrons that are naturally formed as cells turn food into energy. This cellular "exhaust" has been found to speed up the aging process and to raise risk of cardiovascular disease, cancer, and Alzheimer's disease. Antioxidants, which are found in healthy foods and made in the body, can mop up free radicals, but often we don't eat enough antioxidant-rich foods to do this job well.

Consult pages 51–52 in Chapter 3 for more on homocysteine and how to lower it with B vitamin supplements.

tom number) at rest, it needs to be brought down. Diabetics and those with kidney disease are recommended to maintain their blood pressure below 130/80. If you don't do so, you are putting yourself at risk for heart disease and stroke.

In recent years, those with systolic blood pressure between 120 and 139 or diastolic pressure between 80 and 89 have been told that they are "prehypertensive." If this happens to you, don't leap into starting a prescription; first, try exercise, diet, and supplements (more on this later), along with stress-reducing practices.

Here's a review of the classes of medications most commonly prescribed for blood pressure, the nutrients they may deplete, and suggestions for supplementation. Each of the drugs in each of these classes has a long list of potential side effects and interactions. You can find up-to-date drug labeling and side-effect information at www.pdrhealth.com.

If you are taking ACE inhibitors or calcium channel blockers, here's some information you should have: according to a large study carried out by the U.S. government, the newer, more expensive angiotensin-converting enzyme (ACE) inhibitors may not be any more effective than older, much cheaper diuretics. The ALLHAT (Antihypertensive and Lipid-Lowering Treatment to Prevent Heart Attack Trial) concluded that thiazide-type diuretics are better at preventing heart attacks in people at high risk than ACE inhibitors and calcium channel blockers. (High-risk patients are those with diabetes and/or hypertension.) You can read more about this in *Overdosed America: The Broken Promise of American Medicine* by John Abramson, M.D. (Harper Perennial, 2005).

CLASSES OF ANTIHYPERTENSIVES

The sheer volume of antihypertensive medications prohibits me from listing every single one in every class. If you don't see your medications listed here, your pharmacist and medical team should be able to tell you which class your drugs belong to.

THIAZIDE DIURETICS: chlorothiazide (Diuril), chlorthalidone (Hygroton), hydrochlorothiazide (Hydrodiuril), metolazone (Mykrox, Zaroxolyn)

These drugs are usually the first-line therapy for high blood pressure.

Actions: Like all diuretics, they reduce the fluid volume in your body by altering kidney function in a way that flushes out water and salt.

Side effects: Increased frequency of urination.

Nutrients depleted: Thiazide diuretics deplete magnesium, potassium, zinc, sodium, and CoQ_{10}.

Needed supplements: Magnesium (250–500 mg), potassium (100 mg), zinc (25 mg), and CoQ_{10} (100–300 mg).

Caution: Sodium is abundant in most modern diets but if you've been on a sodium-restricted diet, you could run into problems. Speak to your doctor about your adding salt back, in as natural a form as possible, such as sea salt.

LOOP DIURETICS: bumetanide (Burinex), furosemide (Lasix), and torasemide (Torem)

This class of drugs is used to reduce blood pressure.

Actions: These medicines move fluid out of the body, but by a slightly different action on the kidneys.

Side effects: The major side effect with any diuretic is increased frequency of urination.

Nutrients depleted: These drugs deplete calcium, magnesium, potassium, vitamins C, B_1 and B_6, and zinc.

Needed supplements: Take calcium (1,000 mg), magnesium (250–500 mg), potassium (100 mg), vitamins C (1,000 mg), B_1 (320 mg), and B_6 (10–25 mg) and zinc (25 mg).

POTASSIUM-SPARING DIURETICS: amiloride (Midamor), spironolactone (Aldactone), and triamterene (Dyrenium)

Because they preserve levels of the mineral potassium in the body, these medicines may be prescribed alone or with another diuretic to prevent potassium levels from falling too low—a dangerous imbalance called *hypokalemia.*

Actions: Potassium-sparing diuretics reduce blood pressure through actions on the kidneys that increase the amount of urine made in the body.

Side effects: The major side effect with any diuretic is increased frequency of urination.

Nutrients depleted: These drugs deplete calcium, folic acid, vitamin B_6, magnesium, zinc, and CoQ_{10}.

Needed supplements: Take calcium (1,000 mg), folic acid (400 mcg), vitamin B_6 (10–25 mg), magnesium (500–600 mg), zinc (25 mg), and CoQ_{10} (100–300 mg).

CALCIUM CHANNEL BLOCKERS: amlodipine (Norvasc), diltiazem (Cardizem), felodipine (Plendil), idradipine (DynaCirc), nicardipine (Cardene), nisoldipine (Sular), and verapamil (Calan, Covera HS, Isoptin, Veralam)

This drug class reduces blood pressure through a different mechanism than the diuretics.

Actions: These drugs reduce the heart's pumping force and dilate arteries.

Side effects: Possible side effects include headache, edema (swelling) in ankles and feet; verapamil may worsen congestive heart failure or cause constipation.

Nutrients depleted: This drug class can deplete potassium.

Needed supplement: Take 100 mg of potassium.

ANGIOTENSIN CONVERTING ENZYME (ACE) INHIBITORS: captopril (Capoten), enalapril (Vasotec), lisinopril (Prinivil), ramipril (Altace)

ACE inhibitors are a newer class of drugs that are used to treat high blood pressure.

Actions: These drugs block the formation of a blood vessel-constricting chemical called *angiotensin* in the kidneys, as a result, blood pressure is lowered.

Side effects: ACE inhibitors can cause chronic, non-productive cough; reduction of kidney function; and allergic reaction, which can occur at any time while taking the medication.

Nutrient depleted: These medications deplete zinc.

Needed supplement: Take 25 mg of zinc.

ANGIOTENSIN RECEPTOR BLOCKERS (ARBs): candesartan (Atacand), inbesartan (Avapro), losartin (Cozaar), telmisartin (Micardis), and valsartin (Diovan)

Actions: Like ACE inhibitors, ARBs work by dilating blood vessels, making the heart's job easier.

Side effects: Rarely, reduction in kidney function.

Nutrients depleted: None reported.

BETA BLOCKERS: atenolol (Tenormin), metoprolol (Lopressor, Toprol-XL), and propanolol (Inderal)

Beta blockers are one of the oldest and safest classes of antihypertensive drugs. Most of their generic names end in "-lol."

Actions: Lowers blood pressure by reducing the force and speed of the heartbeat. A related class, the alpha-beta blockers, also works by slowing heart rate.

Side effects: Side effects may include excessive heart rate slowing; inability to raise heart rate much during exercise; worsening of congestive heart failure; and rarely, confusion, depression, or worsening erectile dysfunction (impotence).

Nutrient depleted: Beta blockers deplete CoQ_{10} and reduce production of a hormone called melatonin. By blocking beta receptors, these medicines may also block the action of an enzyme needed to make this hormone, which is produced at nightfall and promotes sound sleep.

Needed supplement: Take 100–300 mg of CoQ_{10}.

CENTRALLY ACTING ANTIHYPERTENSIVES: alpha-methyldopa (Aldomet), clonidine (Catapres), and guanfacine (Tenex)

These drugs are less-used alternatives for hypertension than the other classes listed above.

Actions: These drugs act on the nervous system in ways that alter the tension of blood vessel walls—reducing the "fight-or-flight" stimulation from brain to arteries.

Side effects: Because they act on the central nervous system, their side effects can include drowsiness and depression.

Nutrient depleted: These medicines deplete CoQ_{10}.

Needed supplement: Take 100–300 mg of CoQ_{10}.

VASODILATORS: hydralazine (Apresoline), doxazosen (Cardura), and minoxidil (Loniten)

This class of antihypertensives is not used often; you might recognize the minoxidil as the generic name for the hair-growing medicine Rogaine. They are the same chemical, and studies on its use for blood-pressure lowering revealed its usefulness for growing hair on balding heads.

Actions: These drugs reduce blood pressure by acting directly on blood vessel walls to relax them open.

Side effects: Dizziness, headache, and rapid heartbeat (*tachycardia*) are not uncommon—and these side effects are frequent and severe enough to cause doctors to reserve vasodilators only for severe or hard-to-treat hypertension.

Nutrients depleted: These medicines can deplete CoQ_{10} and vitamin B_6.

Needed supplements: Take 100–300 mg of CoQ_{10} and 10–25 mg of vitamin B_6.

NATURAL REMEDIES FOR HYPERTENSION

Some natural remedies work to take blood pressure down a few notches into safe territory.

- *Diet is a big one here!* Stick with the plan I've described in this book, and your blood pressure, cholesterol, and weight are going to come down. The DASH (Dietary Approaches to Stop Hypertension) diet, which is commonly recommended by mainstream docs, will work too, but in my opinion it overemphasizes grains. My recommendations in Chapter 2 resembles the DASH diet in many ways, but I wouldn't advise you to consume six to eight servings of grains per day, and you should avoid refined grains entirely (as in white flour).

- *Reduce stress—by any means necessary.* If you know you need to be less sedentary, and avoid the effects of stress, try meditation, biofeedback, deep breathing, aromatherapy, massage, yoga, or regular exercise, whatever appeals to you. I cannot overstate the importance of having multiple tools to defuse stress, and of working your muscles and cardiovascular system *regularly*—whether you need medications or not.

- *Take herbal supplements and high-powered antioxidants.* Some supplements appear to be effective at lowering blood pressure. See the recommendations at the end of the chapter for a list of specific supplements and dosage recommendations. Check with your pharmacist before adding garlic or hawthorn to your daily supplements.

- *Cram your diet full of antioxidants, anti-inflammatory herbs, and antioxidant-rich foods.* Anyone at risk for heart disease, or who already has been diagnosed with it, should eat plenty of colorful vegetables and fruit, organic if possible, and two or three servings of low-toxin fish (sardines, anchovies, wild-caught salmon) weekly. Avoid margarine and other sources of trans fats. Use olive or macadamia nut oils for cooking. Add herbs and spices with anti-inflammatory, antioxidant punch such as curry powder, turmeric, rosemary, ginger, and garlic to your food as often as possible.

- *Sip green tea once or twice a day.* Try one of the many available varieties of green tea, which has strong antioxidant properties. A glass of red wine once a day is also heart healthy and full of antioxidants, as long as it doesn't interact with your medicines.

- *Eat . . . chocolate?* Dark chocolate has, in recent years, been found to be an excellent source of antioxidants—and may even directly lower blood pressure! Indulge with moderation, since it's the rare occasion when you'll consume chocolate without any sugar to temper its bitterness.

THE CARDIOVASCULAR HEALTH SUPPLEMENT PROGRAM

The recommendations in the multivitamin/mineral program in Chapter 2 are likely to cover you on many of these fronts if you take statins or antihypertensive drugs. You may need to add more of some nutrients to match the dosages listed here for replenishing depletions and improving overall cardiovascular health.

For homocysteine lowering and replenishing B vitamin depletions:

- Folic acid: 400 mcg daily

- Vitamin B_6: 10–25 mg daily

- Vitamin B_{12}: 200 mcg daily

For replenishing depletions from cardiovascular drugs, as well as for improving overall cardiovascular health:

- Calcium: 1,000 mg daily

- CoQ_{10}: 100–300 mg daily

- Magnesium: 250–500 mg daily

- Omega-3 fatty acids (from fish oil): 1,000–3,000 mg of combined EPA and DHA daily

- Potassium: 100 mg daily

- Tocotrienols: 100 mg daily

- Zinc: 25 mg daily

For lowering cholesterol:

- D-ribose: 5 grams, twice daily

- Niacin: Start with 100 mg daily as inositol hexanicotinate or Niaspan and work gradually up to 1.5 to 3 grams; please check with your doctor first!

- Sterols: 1.6–2.4 grams daily, from supplements or sterol-enriched spreads

For lowering high blood pressure:

- Garlic: 1–2 raw cloves of garlic daily or, 1 tablet or capsule containing 300 mg of dried garlic powder (1.3 percent allicin, or 0.6 percent allicin yield) two to three times daily, or 7.2 grams daily of aged garlic extract; garlic also has modest cholesterol-lowering effects

- Grapeseed extract: 100–200 mg daily

- Hawthorn: 1,500 mg daily

- Magnesium: 500–600 mg daily

Note: While antioxidant supplements, like most nutrients, almost never interact with drugs, some herbs with drug-like effects can have risky interactions with prescription medications.

You can often lower your cholesterol and blood pressure with diet, lifestyle, and natural supplements. Then, when medications are necessary, use them with caution, take the lowest dose possible, and make sure to take your supplements to stave off depletion and enjoy the best possible heart health. Next we'll look at anti-inflammatories.

FIVE

Prescriptions for Arthritis: Non-Steroidal Anti-Inflammatory Drugs

nna, my friend's mother, was in amazing health for a woman of eighty-two, her only medical problem being arthritis of the spine and hip. Her doctor prescribed a common anti-arthritic drug, Vioxx.

At that time, *COX-2 inhibitor* drugs like Vioxx and Celebrex, a newer class of *non-steroidal anti-inflammatory drugs* (NSAIDs), were replacing the older NSAIDs like Naprosyn and Aleve, Motrin and Advil, and Voltaren, Athrotec, and Cataflam. The older NSAIDs were known to cause ulcers and internal bleeding, while the new "super aspirins" were supposed to reduce that risk.

One day, Anna suddenly passed out and fell to the floor. She had the presence of mind, when she awoke, to call the paramedics using her Medic Alert pendant. She had begun bleeding from a gastric ulcer. Had help not arrived in time, she would have bled to death.

She complained afterwards, when she was back to her spunky old self, "I thought Vioxx didn't cause that problem—that was why I was spending the big bucks on it instead of the old generic drug I was using before . . . and it didn't even work that well!" I explained to her that these drugs *could* cause those same common NSAID side effects of intestinal ulcers and bleeding—it just didn't happen quite as often.

Only a few months later, the Vioxx cookie crumbled. The drug was found to cause heart attacks in about one in three hundred patients taking it. The Food and Drug Administration (FDA) estimated that between 88,000 and 139,000 heart attacks had been caused, at least in part, by Vioxx—and that 30 to 40 percent had probably been fatal. The drug was voluntarily withdrawn by its manufacturer.

How would a pain medicine cause heart attacks? By affecting enzymes that produce chemicals that help to control inflammation, pain, fever, and other aspects of the immune response. (See pages 61–63 for a more detailed definition of inflammation.)

Older NSAIDs block the activity of two enzymes, COX-1 and COX-2—both of which are involved in the body's production of the chemicals that produce pain and inflammation. However, these chemicals are fabulous multi-taskers. COX-1 also maintains the health of the gastrointestinal (GI) tract lining. This is why blocking it with NSAIDs can cause ulcers and bleeding. Selective COX-2 inhibitors like Vioxx and Celebrex block only COX-2.

Despite drug companies' highest hopes, it turns out that blocking only COX-2 doesn't eliminate the risk of GI bleeding. And, blocking only COX-2 affects the clotting of blood and flexibility of blood vessels in ways that bring about an increased risk of heart disease.

In a nutshell, we know now that the newer COX-2 inhibitors are all likely to increase cardiovascular risk. Since this discovery, many of the older NSAIDS have been implicated in raising heart disease risk as well. This means tough choices for people who need help with arthritis pain or other kinds of muscle or joint pain.

WHAT IS ARTHRITIS?

The word arthritis means "inflammation of the joints" and can include several types. *Osteoarthritis* (OA) is the most common—the kind of arthritis that often afflicts people in the knees, fingers, hips, or back as they age or because of wear and tear. *Rheumatoid arthritis* (RA) is less common, and is an *autoimmune* disease: a disease that can affect the entire body, and that involves out-of-control inflammation. RA affects approximately 2.1 million people in the United States; 75 percent are women. It isn't usually related to aging or wear-and-tear, and tends to strike at a younger age than osteoarthritis. Joints affected by RA inflammation can lose cartilage and end up with OA.

An osteoarthritic joint has lost some or all of the tough, moist, slippery cushion of cartilage that once prevented bone from rubbing against bone. This can happen from overuse, underuse, injury, poor posture, being overweight, or a genetic tendency towards arthritic disease. Food sensitivities or allergies can also contribute to arthritic pain (see inset at right).

As OA progresses, small bits of cartilage can break off and float around in the joint space, causing inflammation and pain. Any joint pain, swelling, or stiffness that lasts for two weeks or more should be evaluated by a doctor; catching the problem early can help minimize damage.

Although it mostly addresses OA, this chapter will cover some anti-inflammatory supplements, including fish oil, that have been found to help with RA as well.

DRUGS FOR ARTHRITIC PAIN: MANY SIDE EFFECTS, DIFFICULT CHOICES

When you are in pain and looking for a way out, you're faced with many choices:

- *Topical creams containing capsaicin.* Capsaicin, also known as *substance P,* is a compound derived from hot peppers. Creams containing it aren't really drugs, but natural medicines that happen to be available on most drugstore shelves among the OTC meds. Smoothing a

Rheumatoid Arthritis and Food Allergy/Sensitivity

Up to twenty percent of RA sufferers get better, while the rest have recurrent problems for the rest of their lives. If you or someone you care about is coping with RA, take note that there is a diet that is very helpful in relieving symptoms. (The same may be true for OA; more on this later.)

Research suggests that people susceptible to RA suffer from "leaky gut." Due to infection or some other problem, the intestinal lining literally develops tiny gaps between the cells, rather than the normally tightly packed cells. This allows larger molecules of food that are not fully broken down to pass through these spaces and into the bloodstream. The immune system does not recognize these normal foods in that form, and sees them as foreign invaders. Doing its job, it then begins to react against these enemies or *antigens,* causing inflammation—which often affects the joints. So, a normal milk or wheat molecule that is not fully broken down can become an antigen, or enemy, and the source of inflammation.

An elimination diet (see page 97) can help people with RA to reduce symptoms and reduce dependency on powerful medications such as methotrexate, etanercept (Enbrel), and corticosteroids. A "Paleolithic diet" that contains no processed food has also been found to be helpful for RA, as have lacto-vegetarian diets (containing no meat or eggs). Anyone interested in learning more about this diet should read *The Paleo Diet* by Loren Cordain, Ph.D. (Wiley, 2002).

capsaicin cream onto painful joints creates heat, which can help soothe pain and muscle tension. Brand names include Capsin, Capzasin-HP Arthritis Formula, Capzasin-P, Dolorac, Menthac Arthritis Cream with Capsaicin, RT Capsin, Salonpas Pain Patch with Capsaicin, Trixaicin, and Zostrix. Be careful not to get these creams in or near your eyes—they'll sting!

- *Acetaminophen (Tylenol).* This drug reduces pain without affecting inflammation. It is implicated in tens of thousands of cases of liver damage, including around 450 deaths, every year, and is the single largest contributing factor to liver failure that requires liver transplants. This drug is included in many multi-drug, over-the-counter (OTC) combinations, and taking even slightly more than the recommended amount can seriously damage your liver. Acetaminophen should never be combined with alcohol, due to their combined effects on the liver. For more serious pain—which usually involves muscular spasms or inflammation:

- *Muscle relaxants like carisoprodol (Soma) or diazepam (Valium).* Drowsiness, dizziness, dry mouth, and addiction are common side effects.

- *Narcotic painkillers* like oxycodone, morphine, codeine, and tramadol hydrochloride (Ultram). Even more intense drowsiness and dizziness are standard with these meds, and addiction is even more likely.

- *Cortisone injections* directly into painful joints. If inflammation sets in with a vengeance, you may be advised to have cortisone injected into the most painful areas. An alternative is injections of *hyaluronic acid,* a building block of healthy cartilage that quite a few of my patients have benefited from. A variation on this is *prolotherapy.* It consists of an injection into the joint of an irritant such as a sugar solution to create more collagen growth, which stabilizes the joint. This can stop the degenerative process and eliminate the pain.

NON-STEROIDAL ANTI-INFLAMMATORY DRUGS

Old-guard NSAIDs include aspirin, naproxen, indomethacin, piroxicam, diclofenac, diflunisal, etodolac, fenoprofen, ketoprofen, ketorolac, meclofenamate, nabumetone, tolmetin, and mefenamic acid. Many (if not all) of these medicines can cause GI ulcers and heart problems. The newest generation of NSAIDs, COX-2 inhibitors such as celecoxib (Celebrex), lumiracoxib (Prexige), valdecoxib (Bextra) are now the most widely used for arthritis. Many of the adverse effects seen with older NSAIDs are also seen with the COX-2 inhibitors—with the likely exception of increased risk of heart problems.

Actions: All NSAIDs block the production of hormone-like substances in the body that produce inflammation and pain.

Side effects: All NSAIDs carry significant risk of gastrointestinal erosion that can lead to GI bleeding. (See "The NSAID Catch-22" on page 86 for more on other adverse effects.)

Nutrients depleted: NSAIDs deplete folate and vitamin C (see below).

Needed supplements: Take 500–1,000 mg of vitamin C and 400–800 mcg of folic acid.

NSAID-INDUCED NUTRIENT DEPLETIONS: FOLATE AND VITAMIN C

Research clearly demonstrates that aspirin and other NSAIDs—including the COX-2 inhibitor Celebrex—deplete folate. Aspirin has also been found to deplete vitamin C. Supplementing with these nutrients while using any NSAID—all of which work by the same general mechanism— is advisable.

The mechanism for folate depletion with these drugs is complex. Basically, the therapeutic effect of these drugs operates through a biochemical mechanism that also depletes folate in the bloodstream. The fall in blood folate levels over only a few days suggests a strong risk of deficiency within a short period in people who take these medications.

Folate intake is often lacking to start with. It's found in whole foods, such as vegetables and whole grains, and most people don't eat nearly enough of those foods. The consequences of folate depletion may include anemia, cervical dysplasia (a precursor to cervical cancer), and high homocysteine. For information on the many roles of folate, and the ways in which depletion can be harmful, turn to the section on Folic Acid/Folate on page 49.

Women who become pregnant while low in folate run the risk of having a baby with serious spinal cord defects. This is why it's recommended that all women of child-bearing age, and especially, those who are pregnant, take 800 micrograms (mcg) of folic acid daily. (Folic acid is the form found in supplements, while folate is found in foods.) Folate is also important for cancer and heart disease prevention. Anyone using NSAIDs on a regular basis should supplement with 400 to 800 mcg of folic acid daily.

NSAIDs also reduce vitamin C levels and activity in the body. We know from several studies that people with OA have lower vitamin C levels in their blood and *synovial fluid* (natural lubrication) in their joints, and are more likely to be deficient than people without OA.

A study from Boston University tracked a group of 640 senior citizens to determine the role of nutrients in osteoarthritis risk. About half started out the study with arthritic symptoms. By the end of the eight-year study, it was evident that those who took in the most vitamin C from food and supplements were *three times less likely* to end up with arthritis or to have worsening symptoms. Joint pain was also much less in those who consumed more vitamin C, a natural anti-inflammatory.

Don't go another day without replenishing it! This nutrient is so important that only a handful of animals—including humans—fail to produce vitamin C in their bodies. Most creatures that produce their own C make the equivalent of a human-sized dose of *10 grams a day*— far more than the measly RDA of 60 milligrams (mg).

The NSAID Catch-22

Another adverse effect of NSAIDs: they inhibit the action of enzymes that are needed to create healthy cartilage. Essentially, this means that the drugs used to relieve arthritis-related discomfort *accelerate the progression of the disease.*

One study of people with knee arthritis found that 47 percent of those taking the NSAID indomethacin got worse, as opposed to only 22 percent of those on placebo. (An interesting note: a lot of other research has shown that the placebo effect, where a "dummy pill" relieves symptoms despite not having any active drug, is especially pronounced in people with arthritis. More on this later.) Another study of 635 people with knee OA found that the NSAID diclofenac—compared with a placebo—more than doubled their risk of developing arthritis in the hip, and more than tripled their risk of getting OA in the other knee. Bottom-line: although they relieve pain, NSAIDs inhibit the creation of new cartilage and speed up its destruction. This seems a poor trade-off!

VITAMIN C: GOOD NUTRITION WHILE USING NSAIDS

Vitamin C (ascorbic acid) is an antioxidant vitamin that also happens to be a building block of *collagen*. Collagen is the material the body uses to build connective tissue, including skin, blood vessel walls, gums, bone, teeth, tendons, ligaments, and cartilage. Depletion of vitamin C could partially explain why NSAIDs cause cartilage to break down. This vitamin "activates" folic acid and is a part of the process of building neurotransmitters and steroid hormones.

The highest concentrations of vitamin C in the body are in the adrenal glands. These walnut-sized glands, which sit above the kidneys, crank out hormones that raise heart rate, breathing rate, and blood pressure in response to stress. When you have an adrenaline rush, you have your adrenals to thank (or curse).

Stress "uses up" vitamin C, and a shortage of vitamin C short-circuits the body's ability to cope with stressful situations. We have plenty of dietary sources, but the vitamin C drain of the hurried/worried modern world makes supplementation important.

Other reasons to appreciate vitamin C:

- People with allergies often find vitamin C works well as a natural antihistamine.

- Supplements of this vitamin may help to reduce asthma symptoms.

- Vitamin C has an anti-inflammatory effect. It promotes the making of anti-inflammatory chemicals and blocks the action of enzymes that promote cartilage-dissolving inflammation.

- Vitamin C plays a role in cardiovascular health. It helps prevent free radicals from oxidizing (or 'rusting') "bad" LDL (low-density lipoprotein) cholesterol, which makes that cholesterol less toxic to the arteries of the heart. Its role in maintaining strong, flexible blood vessel walls further supports heart health.

- Good intake of vitamin C may help prevent varicose veins.

- Vitamin C is a great helpmate for fighting off all kinds of infection. Treating a cold with vitamin C has been found to reduce its duration by 35 percent, and to substantially reduce the intensity of symptoms. I recommend high-dose vitamin C at the first sign of a cold, flu, or other bacterial or viral infections.

    Vitamin C boosts the action of the immune system by increasing the production of white blood cells, antibodies, and the natural antiviral, interferon. Taking 500–1,000 mg of vitamin C every hour or so as soon as symptoms begin will sometimes stop the bug in its tracks— even with really tough viral infections like herpes and shingles.

- For decades, scientists have investigated the use of vitamin C to prevent and even treat cancer. The higher the levels of vitamin C in your body, the lower your risk of gastrointestinal and cervical cancer. Benefit of high vitamin C levels has also been seen in prevention of bladder cancer.

Anyone taking a NSAID should include 1,000–3,000 mg of vitamin C per day in their multinutrient plan. Keep in mind that high doses aren't dangerous—any excess goes out through the urine—but can cause diarrhea, gas, abdominal cramping, or bloating. If you experience these side effects, switch to magnesium or calcium ascorbate, which are buffered (non-acidic) forms of vitamin C. Be consistent; if you use NSAIDs on an ongoing basis, your body needs daily replenishment to ensure that levels remain in an optimal range.

There have been warnings about vitamin C causing kidney stones, but further research has shown this to be untrue. For more information on vitamin C, see my *User's Guide to Vitamin C* (Basic Health Publications, 2003).

OTHER NUTRIENTS AND HERBS FOR PEOPLE WITH OSTEOARTHRITIS

Nutrition can play quite a helpful role in managing your arthritis. Since arthritis is so common, and because standard drug therapies have such serious side effects, there's been a good deal of research into nutritional treatments.

Omega-3 Fatty Acids

DHA and EPA, the omega-3 fats from fish oil, help reduce inflammation and pain, likely just as well as ibuprofen does. They also appear to help build bone and cartilage. In one study, 1,200 to 2,400 mg of DHA/EPA from fish oil was given to OA patients with back and neck pain that could not be fixed surgically. After seventy-five days, 60 percent reported that their joint pain had improved, and 59 percent stopped taking their NSAIDs while on the fish oil. Most said they planned to keep taking the fish oil after the study ended. Omega-3s are so good for you in so many ways—and so deficient in most modern diets—that I recommend them to everyone.

Dose: Start out with 1 to 2 grams a day (1,000 to 2,000 mg) of fish oil. Use a brand that guarantees that it is free from mercury and other toxins. Smaller fish are less contaminated since they are lower on the food chain. Larger fish accumulate more toxins. If you end up with fish burps, use enteric-coated capsules that dissolve only when they are past the stomach, in the small intestine.

Vitamin D

Studies show that low levels of the "sunshine vitamin" correlate with increased symptoms of arthritis. People with joint and muscle pain often get some relief with vitamin D supplementation. This nutrient is essential, too, in the prevention of osteoporosis.

Dose: Take 1,000 international units (IU) a day, or more if blood tests show a serious deficiency.

Glucosamine/Chondroitin

Both of these substances are *glycosaminoglycans* (GAGs), building materials for making cartilage. Using both together can reduce pain and promote joint healing in arthritis—with pain relief benefits rivaling those of the NSAIDs, without those drugs' liabilities.

In the biggest study on the subject, a $12.5 million study performed by the National Institutes of Health, 67 percent of 1,583 participants who took both glucosamine (1,500 mg) and chondroitin (1,200 mg) daily had reduced pain. (Keep in mind that 60 percent of the participants who took a placebo also reported a reduction in pain—a testament to the power of the placebo effect!) A separate analysis of participants who had moderate to severe pain found an enhanced effect of the glucosamine/chondroitin (pain reduction in 79.2 percent) combination over the placebo (pain reduction in 54.3 percent).

Dose: Start with 1,500 mg of glucosamine plus 1,200 mg of chondroitin, or start out with glucosamine only, adding chondroitin only if you don't feel benefits within about three months' time.

Boswellia serrata

Boswellia is a traditional Ayurvedic medicinal herb. It has been used to relieve arthritic symptoms for thousands of years. Modern research has pitted *Boswellia* against NSAIDs and found that it may be a more effective anti-inflammatory than the drugs. It works through at least three different mechanisms to reduce inflammation, and seems especially useful for rheumatoid arthritis and other types of arthritis where inflammation is a major component.

Dose: Take a supplement that contains 600 mg per day of boswellic acids, the herb's active constituent.

Ginger

Throughout history, ginger has been used to reduce inflammation and arthritis pain, soothe digestive upsets, and clear up chest congestion. Like *Boswellia,* ginger acts as a natural NSAID, with a broader enzyme-blocking action than anti-inflammatory drugs. Ginger also contains many antioxidant compounds. "In vitro" (test-tube) research and "in vivo" studies (using animals and people) find that consuming ginger most often successfully reduces inflammation and pain.

Dose: Consume ginger as part of your diet and supplement with up to 4 grams per day of powdered ginger.

Turmeric/Curcumin

Indian food is well seasoned with turmeric, a pungent yellow member of the ginger family that is an excellent natural anti-inflammatory. The key active ingredient in this spice is curcumin, which gives turmeric its distinctive yellow color. Turmeric is also a potent antioxidant and helps to kill bacteria. It has no side effects.

Dose: Use curry powder liberally in foods—try it in chicken salad!—and supplement with 400–600 mg of turmeric, three times a day.

MSM (Methylsulfonylmethane)

MSM is a form of sulfur, which is a building block of cartilage and other connective tissue. In this form, sulfur is a mild anti-inflammatory and has been found to help relieve arthritis pain. A study published in 2005 found that a combination of glucosamine (see above) and MSM were more effective, more quickly, than either one alone. Even separately, both significantly relieved OA pain. Another study of MSM alone, this one from 2006, enrolled fifty men and women aged forty to seventy-six, all of whom had knee OA. They got either 3 grams of MSM daily or a placebo twice a day for twelve weeks. The MSM reduced pain and improved function significantly more than the placebo, with no negative side effects.

Dose: Take up to 6 grams daily of MSM.

Bromelain

Bromelain is an enzyme found in fresh pineapple. It has anti-inflammatory and pain-relieving effects, and has been studied widely as a natural therapy for OA.

Dose: Take 200–400 mg per day, between meals. (If you take it during meals, it gets used up digesting your food.)

Avocado/Soybean Unsaponifiables (ASU)

ASU is an extract of fatty acids from avocado and soybeans. No matter how many avocadoes or blocks of tofu you manage to swallow, you can't match the fatty acid composition of ASU; its so-called *unsaponifiables* make up only 1/1000th of its total fatty acid content.

ASU has anti-inflammatory effects and appears to help repair cartilage. At this writing, there's a lot of excitement over studies that show ASU to be effective in reducing knee and hip OA stiffness and pain. In France, ASU is a prescription medicine; in the United States, it's catching on a lot more slowly.

Dose: Start with 300 mg per day, and give it up to two months to reduce your symptoms.

Devil's Claw (*Harpagophytum procumbens*)

This African herb has been shown to be effective for the majority of people with low back, knee, or hip pain. Devil's claw seems to do its work by reducing inflammation.

In one study, 250 men and women with low back, hip, or knee pain took a devil's claw extract containing 60 mg of total *harpagoside* (the herb's active ingredient). After taking the extract daily for eight weeks, between 50 and 70 percent noted some improvement in pain, with an average reduction in reported pain of 30 to 40 percent. Younger people tended to have more noticeable pain relief than older people. Only twenty-nine people (11.6 percent) reported adverse effects that could possibly be attributed to the medication, including digestive upset, nausea, vomiting, and allergic rash.

Dose: Take 60 mg daily.

EXERCISE: A NEW PERSPECTIVE ON OSTEOARTHRITIS PAIN

Of course, anyone with arthritis should be engaged in regular exercise. It's very common for an arthritic joint to become worse for lack of movement as muscles weaken and the joint becomes less and less stable. Your doctor should be able to set you up with appropriate physical therapy and a gentle exercise program that keeps your joints as supple as possible and the muscles that support them strong.

Think you couldn't possibly exercise through your arthritis pain? Although arthritis is a leading cause of disability, it's not always painful. Surprisingly, x-ray findings of arthritic damage to joints are a poor predictor of the amount of pain experienced by the person being x-rayed. In other words, one person with badly damaged joints may have no pain at all, while another with minimal damage—or even no damage at all—may be debilitated by pain.

"Sure, great," you might be saying, "but I'm in pain. Are you saying it's all in my head?!?" Absolutely not. Your pain is real—but many factors influence your perception of pain, from your balance of amino acids or minerals (low levels of serotonin or magnesium can increase pain perception), plus your thoughts, emotions, beliefs, and fears.

John Sarno, M.D., is a physician and New York University professor of Rehabilitation Medicine. He has written several books about the mysteries of muscle, joint, and skeletal pain: why it's so much worse for some than others, what causes it, and what can be done to heal it. Dr. Sarno has coined the term tension myositis syndrome (TMS) to describe symptoms of pain that can't be traced back to a specific cause. Here's where the concept of the pain being "all in your head" has some merit.

Dr. Sarno believes that much of the low back pain people suffer is caused by muscular tension in the body clamping down on blood vessels and reducing circulation to the painful body part. That's TMS.

Anyone who's seen a scary movie knows that being afraid translates into a physical response. Thoughts can dramatically alter your body. It's no surprise, then, that pushing down emotions or thoughts can change you physically. Dr. Sarno, in his medical practice, found that nearly 90 percent of people with low back pain had other problems—eczema, heartburn, irritable bowel syndrome, spastic colon, frequent urination—that are believed to be linked to nervous tension, and that's when he began to develop the TMS concept and ways to relieve it.

What's the solution? A process where the person in pain allows him or herself to be aware of the feelings that TMS is helping him or her to avoid. Acceptance of those feelings will then interrupt the cycle of pain and tension. This approach can work for any kind of pain—as long as you are willing to understand and ultimately accept that your pain is being caused by your tension.

Dr. Sarno's work has brought relief to a lot of people with OA, low back pain, disc problems, sciatica, pinched nerve, thoracic outlet syndrome, bursitis, tendonitis, knee pain, elbow pain, fibromyalgia, carpal tunnel syndrome, temporal mandibular joint syndrome (TMJ), and pain in the wrists, hands, lower legs, or feet, as well as unexplained chronic pain. I highly recommend looking at one of his books and applying his advice to yourself. (See the Resources section for his book titles.)

The worst that could happen: you'll be in less pain and more in touch with your deepest thoughts and feelings.

THE HEALTHY JOINT SUPPLEMENT PROGRAM

To replace depletions from NSAIDs, as well as addressing the underlying deficiencies and inflammation, you can take the following supplements as needed.

- Folic acid: 400–800 mcg per day
- Vitamin C: 500–1,000 mg per day

Other helpful supplements:

- Avocado/soybean unsaponifiables (ASU): 300 mg daily (allow up to two months to see results)
- Boswellic acids: 600 mg daily
- Bromelain: 200–400 mg daily, between meals
- Devil's claw: 60 mg daily

- Fish oil: 1–2 grams (1,000–2,000 mg) daily

- Ginger: Up to 4 grams daily in powdered form, or eat it in foods

- Glucosamine/chondroitin: 1,500 mg of glucosamine sulfate per day alone to start; if you don't discern any benefit within three months, try adding 1,200 mg of chondroitin daily

- MSM: Up to 6 grams daily

- Turmeric: 400–600 mg three times daily

Don't forget to follow the diet and multivitamin recommendations from Chapter 2. All forms of arthritis respond well to natural treatments, including supplements. Most of these treatments are side-effect free, and they *treat the problem at its root cause* rather than simply addressing the symptoms. Even if you are taking anti-inflammatories, a good diet and supplement program will begin the healing process.

SIX

Prescriptions for Digestive Function: Drugs for Acid Reflux, Heartburn, and Constipation

mericans have an enormous dependency on over-the-counter (OTC) and prescription drugs for digestive problems. We spend more than $1.2 billion annually on OTC antacids and acid-blocking drugs to treat heartburn, and about $800 million on laxatives. Many of these medicines have nutrient-depleting effects.

Neither the squelching of stomach acid nor drug-induced bowel movements address the root causes of these problems. As you'll see in this chapter, reliance on these kinds of medicines to squash symptoms often ends up worsening the root problem. In the bargain, users of these drugs can end up dependent on them for seemingly "normal" function, even as their bodies' stores of important nutrients needed for *truly* normal, healthy function are drained away.

FOOD MAY BE THE SOURCE OF YOUR MISERY— AND YOUR RETURN TO HEALTH

Modern medicine often ignores the obvious role of processed, adulterated foods and specific food sensitivities in causing many common gastrointestinal (GI) ills. On the other hand, physicians are often faced with patients who aren't willing to change what they're eating, even when told how big a difference this will make in their health.

George weighs 350 pounds, smokes, and drinks several sodas a day. He has long suffered from heartburn or acid reflux. Now, he can likely get rid of this by changing his diet, dropping 100 pounds, quitting his nicotine habit, and drinking water instead of Coca-Cola. Instead, he says to his doctor, "Thanks for the advice. Can I have my prescription now?" This is a scenario faced by most physicians several times a day, year after year. It's no wonder so many docs just pull out the prescription pad rather than aggressively insisting on lifestyle change.

In this chapter, I hope to drive home to you a singular message: *the foods you eat are probably the cause of your distress. Changing your diet is almost sure to cure you.* This can't be said about many health problems—that you have an extraordinary amount of control over your recovery. Such changes may not be simple or easy, but the reward is worth it: relief from chronic heartburn, acid reflux, and constipation.

YOU AREN'T WHAT YOU EAT—YOU ARE WHAT YOU *ABSORB*

The rewards of great digestive health go well beyond relief of symptoms. Your digestive tract is the starting place of the process where the foods you consume are transformed into *you*. Think of it as the place where building materials are sorted out and transported into your body; if the sorting and transport go well, construction runs smoothly, and your body gets built stronger and is more resistant to aging and disease. Optimizing digestive function can give you abundant energy, clearer thinking, more luminous skin, a more youthful appearance, and greater protection against disease.

Simply swallowing a food—even a healthy food—does not ensure that you will be well nourished. It has to be broken down first (in the mouth, stomach, and small intestine), and then absorbed properly (in the small and large intestines), to do its job. For starters, you need to chew your food *thoroughly*, until it's liquid in your mouth, to mix it with salivary enzymes that begin the digestive process. How often do you catch yourself wolfing down your food, barely chewing it, because you're in a rush or just because it's your habit?

Slow down! Chew and chew and chew. The more you chew, the clearer the message to your stomach to begin secreting acid and enzymes to further break down your food. This paves the way for further digestion in the small intestine, where nutrients are absorbed into the bloodstream. More nutrients are absorbed and produced in the large intestine. All of these actions require specific nutrients, and are supported or handicapped by the food choices you make.

Without the proper enzymes and a well-functioning intestinal wall, you may be eating a diet fit for a king, but you'll be malnourished. Your body will become fertile ground for the development of disease.

Poor digestion, in other words, can be at the root of many nutrient depletions, which can cause chronic health conditions. Ironically, the drugs used to treat those chronic health conditions can, in turn, make the depletions even worse. More drugs are added to your regimen. More depletions ensue, and the vicious cycle continues.

THE ELIMINATION DIET

Making the necessary adjustments for better digestive function may not seem easy at first. The most fundamental changes are those described in Chapter 2: they involve getting the junk food, processed food, flour, and sugars out of your life, and making vegetables, lean protein, nuts, and fruit the mainstays of your diet.

Identifying foods or ingredients that you're sensitive to—most commonly, wheat, dairy, soy, peanuts, chocolate, fish, shellfish, corn, yeast, and eggs—may be key for fixing your digestive symptoms at their source. Keeping a food journal and tracking your symptoms will help you to identify food sensitivities and act accordingly. The best way to do this is an "elimination diet." You remove the top allergens (wheat, dairy, sugar, alcohol, and caffeine) for a week and observe how you feel. You then reintroduce them one at a time, and see whether your symptoms return.

I've had amazed patients see their heartburn, constipation, rashes, headaches, back pain, and a myriad of other issues disappear once the offending food was removed, only to return when that food was reintroduced. That was enough to keep them eating "clean" from then on. This same exercise can be used in treating any number of troublesome conditions, including arthritis.

Taking action as soon as symptoms show up will help to prevent them from progressing to a chronic condition. But it's true that some people require GI drugs to have a semblance of normal function. If this describes you, you can still take the steps recommended in this book, and to replace nutrients depleted by your medicines.

Now let's take a look at the medicines used to treat a common gastro-intestinal condition referred to as heartburn, acid reflux, or GERD (gastroesophageal reflux) and the nutrients it can deplete. Throughout the chapter, I will outline the possible causes of these conditions, and how diet and natural remedies can be used instead of OTC and prescription drugs.

HEARTBURN AND ACID REFLUX: ACID GONE WILD?

Corinne was one of the 15 million Americans—that's one in eighteen—who had an episode or more of heartburn *every day*. (Over 60 million

Americans are believed to have it at least once a month.) This forty-three-year-old mother of four tried chewing aluminum-containing antacids and cutting down on spicy foods and coffee, but nothing seemed to help.

She turned to the OTC acid-reducer Zantac, and felt some relief from the heartburn—but her stomach became bloated and full for hours after each meal, and the constipation that started while she was popping several antacids a day grew worse. Her husband informed her that her breath was "stinky," which didn't surprise her. When she swallowed, she felt like something was caught in her throat.

A dry cough finally sent her to her doc, who told her that all of her symptoms, including her cough, sounded a lot like GERD. Repeated exposure of her esophagus to acid from her stomach was causing inflammation and irritation. He warned her that untreated GERD could lead to permanent damage, and maybe even to a precancerous condition called Barrett's esophagus. She left with a prescription for another acid-lowering drug called Prevacid that, according to her doctor, she would probably have to take for the rest of her life.

Corinne wasn't too thrilled about this. Her family was on a fixed income and didn't have health insurance. This really set her stomach acid churning—but, as it turned out, she didn't have much of it to churn. You see, too much stomach acid wasn't Corinne's problem in the first place—it was *too little* stomach acid.

She learned this after she came to see me and I conducted a special test called a *Heidelberg Test*. To her surprise, Corinne turned out to be *hypo*chlorhydric—not making adequate stomach acid. When I told her, she was incredulous. "How can I have been burning my esophagus when I don't have enough acid?"

The Acid Reflux Paradox

Your stomach makes hydrochloric acid (HCl) and enzymes that, along with the powerful muscular churning of the stomach wall, breaks the foods you eat into a sort of "soup" called *chyme*. That chyme has to reach a certain level of acidity before it can pass into the small intestine. When food remains in your stomach too long, the stomach "burps" some of it back up into the esophagus, causing a burning sensation. Bottom-line: lowering acid production can, paradoxically, increase your risk of heartburn and reflux.

Ten to fifteen percent of Americans are hypochlorhydric, and about *half* of people over sixty don't make enough acid to properly break down their food, giving them heartburn. Because the symptoms are the same as those of *too much* stomach-acid production, they tend to be treated with acid-reducing drugs.

Low stomach acid reduces your body's ability to extract nutrients from food. Further suppressing and buffering acids with antacids worsen this problem, leading to malnutrition. Both low acid levels and acid-reducing drugs reduce the stomach's production of *intrinsic factor,* which is needed for the absorption of vitamin B_{12}. Research has shown a link between antacid use and memory loss with aging, and B_{12} lack is believed to be the reason for this.

Bottom-line: long-term use of drugs to buffer and reduce digestive acids could substantially affect your body's levels of important nutrients—even if you weren't hypochlorhydric at the start.

Keep in mind that some people *do* make too much stomach acid. For these people, supplementing with extra nutrients, as recommended later in this chapter, will help, as will acid-lowering drugs in some cases. For these people, medication to lower acid may be a necessary part of healing or prevention of ulcers.

The most common treatments for heartburn and GERD are drugs that either 1) neutralize acids, as with OTC antacid drugs like Tums; or 2) reduce the action of the stomach's acid-producing machinery. An excellent book on this topic is Dr. Sherry Rogers' *No More Heartburn* (Kensington, 2000).

Helicobacter pylori (H. pylori)

A common cause of heartburn, indigestion, ulcers, and stomach cancer is a bacteria called *Helicobacter pylori. H. pylori* is the only bacterial organism in the stomach that cannot be killed by hydrochloric acid. The 'antacid' effect of *Helicobacter pylori* fools your stomach into producing more acid, and damage to the stomach is the likely result.

According to the U.S. Centers for Disease Control and Prevention (CDC), nine out of ten cases of peptic ulcer disease are caused by infection with *Helicobacter pylori* bacteria. Antibiotic treatment is not always effective, since *H. pylori* is already resistant to any single dose of antibiotics and is often resistant to the commonly prescribed triple and quadruple therapies. However, natural remedies such as mastic and zinc-carnosine (more on these later) have cleared many cases that I've treated over the years, even with no medication at all.

OTC AND PRESCRIPTION DRUGS
FOR HEARTBURN AND ACID REFLUX

There are a slew of OTC and prescription medicines available for treating these conditions; some are quite powerful.

ANTACIDS: aluminum-magnesium mixtures (Di-Gel, Gaviscon, Gelusil, Maalox, Mylanta), and calcium carbonate (Caltrate, Dicarbosil, Rolaids, Titralac, Tums)

These are salts of aluminum, magnesium, or calcium, designed to buffer stomach acid. They are taken either before or after a meal.

Actions: These antacids work in the stomach to neutralize and reduce stomach acid.

Side effects: They commonly cause constipation.

Nutrients depleted: Aluminum-containing antacids appear to be the worst culprits in this drug class when it comes to nutrient depletion. They deplete phosphorus, zinc, vitamins B_{12} and D, and calcium. They have been linked to higher risk of osteoporosis. Calcium-containing antacids can (rarely) cause high calcium levels in the blood (hypercalcemia), which is very dangerous. Lowered stomach acid also can decrease folic acid absorption.

Needed supplements: Calcium (1,000–1,200 mg), folic acid (400 mcg), phosphorus (700 mg), vitamin B_{12} (200 mcg), vitamin D (600–1,000 IU), and zinc (25–50 mg)

H2 BLOCKERS: cimetidine (Tagamet), famotidine (Pepcid), nizatidine (Axid), and ranitidine (Zantac)

These medicines are available both OTC in lower doses and by prescription in higher doses. They block the production of acid in the stomach. They are also used to help the healing of stomach ulcers. Don't use an OTC H2 blocker to treat your own heartburn for more than two weeks without checking in with your doctor.

Actions: These medicines block the production of histamine, a chemical made by the body that triggers the stomach cells to produce acid.

Side effects: Famotidine and ranitidine sometimes cause headache.

Cimetidine interacts with a long list of drugs, including the anti-clotting medicine warfarin (Coumadin), the seizure drug phenytoin (Dilantin), and a seldom-used asthma drug called theophylline (Theo-Dur).

Nutrients depleted: These drugs, like those used to treat type 2 diabetes, deplete levels of vitamin B_{12}. Like antacids, they deplete calcium; and they are also believed to deplete bone-building, cancer-preventive vitamin D.

Needed supplements: Calcium (1,000–1,200 mg), vitamin B_{12} (200 mcg), and vitamin D (600–1,000 IU).

Acid Blockers and Pneumonia

Several studies have shown that the use of acid-suppressing drugs—including H2-blockers and proton pump inhibitors—is linked to increased risk of a certain type of pneumonia. Why would this be?

Stomach acid kills off bacteria, viruses, and other microorganisms that could cause dangerous infections if allowed to pass further into the body. Suppressing acid production, then, reduces this natural bodily defense against hazardous "bugs."

PROTON PUMP INHIBITORS (PPIs): omeprazole (Prilosec, HK-20, Zegerid), esomeprazole (Nexium), lansoprazole (Prevacid, Zoton, Inhibitol), pantoprazole (Protonix, Somac, Pantoloc, Protium), and rabeprazole sodium (Aciphex, Rabecid, Pariet)

These drugs are the most potent of the acid-reducing medications. They reduce stomach acid production by up to 99 percent, using a slightly different mechanism than the H2 blockers. As you might imagine, this big reduction can strongly interfere with nutrient absorption.

Actions: These drugs reduce stomach acid secretion by reducing the action of proton pumps, which are part of the stomach lining's acid-making machinery.

Side effects: Common side effects can include headache, nausea, diarrhea, abdominal pain, dizziness, rash, itching, flatulence, or constipation . . . and increased risk of osteoporosis over the long haul.

A study of 135,000 people fifty and older found that high doses of PPIs, used for a year or more, are just over 2.5 times more likely to break a hip than those who didn't take these drugs at all. Smaller doses raised risk less, to about 1.5 times the risk of non-users. The longer the period of use, the more the risk of fracture rose. This heightened risk of osteoporosis is probably due to the drastic drop in calcium absorption that occurs with these drugs. Some experts believe that the drug itself may hamper the body's ability to build new bone.

Nutrients depleted: B_{12} depletion is listed as a side effect that may occur with long-term use. Calcium absorption is reduced by these drugs as well.

Needed supplements: Calcium (1,000–1,200 mg) and vitamin B_{12} (200 mcg).

NATURAL TREATMENTS FOR HYPOCHLORHYDRIA

If you stop your antacid medication too quickly, you will likely have rebound *hyper*acidity, and you then will have too much acid to thank for your heartburn.

I ended up recommending to Corinne that she change to an OTC histamine blocker, like Zantac or Tagamet. She followed my advice to first take the maximum dose, then gradually wean off until there were no symptoms present. At the same time, we addressed the root cause: her diet. I advised her to avoid processed foods, especially sugars and grains, both of which break down into sugar in the body, interfering with the friendly bacteria in the GI tract. I added in some specific nutrients as well, as follows:

- *Omega-3 fatty acids*.

- *A high-quality probiotic*.

- *Plenty of water* throughout the day—at least eight glasses of pure water.

- *Zinc-carnosine*, a specific combination molecule that has both antibacterial and healing effects on the lining of the stomach and esophagus. It relieves stomach pain, heals ulcers, and may even prevent ulcers by sticking to the stomach wall, where it creates a barrier against stomach acids. Zinc-carnosine also inhibits the growth of *H. pylori*. In a Japanese study, twenty-five patients whose ulcers were confirmed by endoscopy (a test using a telescope that looks at the stomach lining) were given 75 mg of zinc-carnosine twice daily for eight weeks. Stomach pains were relieved in 53.3 percent of the patients after meals, 76.9 percent when fasting, and 90.9 percent at night. At the end of the eight weeks, 65 percent of them were healed of their gastric ulcers—without suppressing the production of acid.

- *Mastic gum*, the sap of the Mediterranean plant *Pistacia lentiscus*, has been used to treat stomach problems for centuries.

The happy ending? Corinne's heartburn was gone for good. You can have the same successful outcome with the right diet and supplement program. Refer to the end of the chapter for a more concise list of the supplements and dosages that can keep you off of acid-reducing drugs— or, if you do need them, that can help restore nutrients depleted by those drugs.

CONSTIPATION NATION

Mass-media health publications often warn of the hazards of "intestinal toxicity." There is some truth to this. With the typical American diet and lack of exercise, elimination can become sluggish, and this can lead to a decline in health as bacteria and yeast multiply in the colon.

When "bad" bacteria and yeasts have overwhelmed "good" bacteria, we're looking at *dysbiosis*. This shift in the natural balance of the colon does indeed create toxic byproducts, and these can be reabsorbed into the body through the colon wall. Those "good" probiotic bacteria also produce nutrients, such as B vitamins, including vitamin B_{12}, that are then absorbed through the wall of the colon and into the body; in a state of dysbiosis, these probiotics may not be able to produce enough of these nutrients to maintain health.

You should have one easy, comfortable bowel movement a day, with a soft texture and about (yes) two feet in total length. You should be able to sit down and comfortably eliminate when the urge strikes you. And the smell shouldn't be too totally awful for you to sit there with it—if it is, then chances are good that there's some dysbiosis going on in there.

In one study, 12 percent of nearly 14,000 people on four continents reported that they suffer from constipation. About a third of people who treat themselves do so with *contact laxatives*, which work by enhancing the contractions of the large intestine to move what's in there out of the body.

If you do require a little help from time to time:

- *Contact laxatives*—also known as stimulant laxatives—are a viable option. Generic, OTC versions include bisacodyl, senna, castor oil, and cascara sagrada (the latter three are actually natural plant-derived medicines that have been used for this purpose for centuries).

But using stimulant laxatives daily or almost daily can backfire on you as your body becomes dependent on this outside stimulation.

- *Hyperosmotic laxatives*, which work by drawing more water into the colon to make bowel movements softer, are also okay for occasional use. But chronic use of any kind of laxative—as is sometimes seen in eating disorders—can be a drain on your nutrient reserves, particularly minerals (calcium, magnesium, potassium) and B vitamins. Types include milk of magnesia, magnesium oxide, and Epsom salts. You can also occasionally take 1,000 to 2,000 mg of magnesium oxide (a cheap form of magnesium used to make supplements) for strong overnight laxative action.

- *Bulk-producing laxatives* are safe and won't cause nutrient depletion. Psyllium, oat bran, ground flaxseeds, and methylcellulose are all bulk-producing. If you decide to use these, it's crucial to use them with the recommended amount of water—and perhaps, a little extra. Without adequate fluid, the bulk can just clog you up more. Some people find that this kind of laxative simply doesn't do the trick for them.

- *Stool softeners and surfactant laxatives* aren't great choices; they work by lubricating the pipes, so to speak, with oils that allow more slippery passage of bowel contents. The body quickly develops tolerance to these kinds of laxatives.

- *Enemas* are also okay occasionally, but repeated use can cause mineral depletion, imbalance of "good" probiotic bacteria in the colon, and loss of the natural responsiveness of the colon.

- *Mineral oil*, a petroleum derivative, acts as an intestinal lubricant. It also coats food particles as well as the lower intestinal walls, mechanically interfering with nutrient absorption. It depletes the fat-soluble vitamins A, D, E, and K, as well as beta-carotene, calcium, and phosphorus. It should not be combined with stool softeners, which may increase its absorption into the body—not good, since mineral oil is toxic when taken internally.

PRESCRIPTIONS FOR CHRONIC CONSTIPATION

Chronic constipation may be the doctor's diagnosis when you have, for three or more months over the last twelve, had three or fewer bowel movements a week; bloating; hard stools; and a feeling that the colon never empties all the way. Many prescription drugs can cause constipation, and sometimes this side effect is treated with drugs to relieve the constipation. For a listing of these drugs, see the inset at right.

There are a few prescription medications used to treat chronic constipation, including lactulose (brand name Enulose), polyethylene glycol (Miralax), and tegaserod (Zelnorm). In March 2007, the Food and Drug Administration (FDA) halted the sale of Zelnorm as a result of safety concerns when research showed that it significantly increased risk of heart attacks, strokes, angina, and death. Quite a price to pay for a constipation medication!

> **Drugs That May Cause Constipation**
>
> - Pain medications (especially narcotics)
> - Antacids that contain aluminum
> - Antispasmodic drugs (given for gastrointestinal cramping or diarrhea)
> - Antidepressant drugs
> - Tranquilizers
> - Iron supplements
> - Anticonvulsants for epilepsy
> - Drugs for Parkinson's disease
> - Calcium channel blockers (given to treat high blood pressure)

These products work mostly by helping to retain water in the stool. None are recommended for any more than short-term use, and can cause diarrhea, nausea, and black, tarry stools. They may deplete some nutrients—any drug that causes diarrhea or nausea can have broad depleting and dehydrating effects—but at this writing, there are no known depletions.

GOOD NUTRITION WHILE USING DIGESTIVE DRUGS

You've seen that several of these medicines deplete B vitamins, particularly B_{12} and folate. When these vitamins are depleted, body levels of homocysteine—a toxic amino acid—rise, and over time this contributes to serious problems such as heart disease, stroke, hypertension, and Alzheimer's disease. The potential hazards of B_{12} and folate depletion and the rise in homocysteine that can result are covered in detail on pages 48–52. Please refer to those pages to discover in more detail why B vitamin supplements are a good idea for anyone using medicines that deplete those vitamins.

The other depletions of concern here are the minerals calcium, zinc, and iron, and vitamin D.

Calcium

Aluminum antacids, H2 blockers, and PPIs decrease calcium absorption from food. Calcium is the most abundant mineral in the body, with the average male body containing 2.5 to 3 pounds and the average female body containing about 2 pounds of calcium. All but 1 percent of that calcium is stored in bones and teeth; the rest has roles in the passage of nutrients and wastes in and out of cells, and in the contraction and relaxation of muscle cells—particularly, those that make up the heart. It follows that adequate calcium helps to keep heart rate regular.

A lack of calcium is a well-known risk factor for osteoporosis. Low calcium is also associated with hypertension—that is, people with low levels of calcium are more likely to have high blood pressure. Colon cancer risk is also increased when calcium is low, and the use of calcium supplements has been found to lower that risk.

Organic dairy products, broccoli, leafy greens, beans, and nuts can help you to meet your daily calcium requirements. Using a supplement is advisable, though. If you take more than your body needs, the excess will be flushed out in your urine. The RDA is 1,000 mg per day; I recommend 1,000 to 1,200 mg daily, along with 500 to 600 mg of magnesium. Zinc (and, sometimes, iron; see below) supplements should also be used; a high dose of calcium without other balancing minerals can end up depleting your absorption of those balancing minerals even further.

Take your calcium and other mineral supplements as far from your acid-reducing medications as possible, for better absorption.

Dose: 1,000–1,200 mg calcium and 500 mg of magnesium.

Zinc

This mineral plays a role in hundreds of enzyme reactions in the body. It is needed to make protein and DNA, and for the detoxification actions of the liver. The immune system uses zinc in many of its most important defenses against disease and in the healing of wounds and skin conditions. Thyroid hormones, which regulate metabolism (the rate at which body cells burn food for energy), rely on zinc-dependent enzymes to convert an inactive form to an active form of hormone. Men need plenty of zinc for prostate health.

H2 blockers deplete this mineral. It's believed that many Americans are borderline zinc deficient, drugs or no drugs, and even a small depletion can compound a preexisting deficiency. Symptoms of low zinc include acne, slow wound healing, menstrual problems, joint pain, poor immunity, light sensitivity, skin problems, and lackluster, brittle hair.

Food sources include seafood (especially oysters), lean meat, liver, eggs, and whole-grain breads and cereals.

Dose: Use a supplement that brings 25–50 mg of zinc into your system daily if you use H2 blockers.

Iron

H2 blockers and antacids deplete this mineral. Others at risk, or who might have increased risk beyond that created by GI medications:

- Women who are still menstruating regularly are at the greatest risk of starting out deficient in iron. Deficiency is less common in post-menopausal women and men, who don't lose iron each month.

- Vegetarians, adolescent girls, people who have bleeding ulcers, and pregnant women are all at increased risk for iron deficiency.

- People with hypochlorhydria are also at risk, as they don't absorb iron from foods very well.

- Chronic use of laxatives or inflammatory diseases of the colon (Crohn's disease, ulcerative colitis) may also increase iron needs.

- People who take nonsteroidal anti-inflammatory drugs (NSAIDs) and have intestinal bleeding may also become iron deficient.

A lack of iron will make you feel tired, because it's a building block for *hemoglobin*, the molecule that carries oxygen around in the bloodstream. Inadequate iron will lead to anemia, where not enough hemoglobin is available to distribute oxygen adequately. Iron deficiency may also cause you to lose your hair or cause you to have a headache. You may start to catch every bug that comes around and get infections more easily. Brittle nails are also a sign of iron deficiency. Like zinc, iron is a part of many essential enzyme reactions. It is needed for good immune system function and for the liver's ability to get rid of toxic substances.

Food sources of iron include liver, organ meats, fish, poultry, dried beans, vegetables, and whole grains. Consult with your doctor if you have iron-deficiency symptoms; he or she may recommend a higher dose. If you are male or a postmenopausal woman and have risk factors for heart disease (or you know you have heart disease), you should avoid iron supplements unless you test out to be deficient; confer with your doctor on this, too.

Caution: Keep all iron supplements away from children. An adult iron supplement can kill a child under the age of five.

Dose: If you use H2 blockers or antacids regularly, it's wise to supplement with 15 mg per day—an amount that can be found in most multi-vitamin/mineral supplements.

Vitamin D

Vitamin D is reduced in the body by H2 blockers. This vitamin works hand-in-hand with calcium and phosphorus, minerals needed for bone health. It also promotes good immune function and helps prevent cancer. Because it's also important for good mood, a detailed description of this vitamin appears in the chapter on antidepressants. See page 125 to learn more about this nutrient.

Dose: Take 600–1,000 mg daily, or more if tests show you are deficient.

OTHER SUPPLEMENTS AND DIET CHANGES TO CONSIDER

Gastrointestinal health and healing can be promoted by taking the following steps.

To Prevent Heartburn and Acid Reflux:

- Drink 8 ounces of water with one tablespoon of apple cider vinegar about thirty minutes before each meal.

- Drink 8 ounces of room-temperature water right after a meal.

- Sleep with the head of your bed elevated by about four inches.

- Stop smoking.

- Keep alcohol consumption to one glass of wine or beer a day.

- Take digestive enzymes with each meal. Use a mixed blend of amylase, lipase, and protease enzymes that help to break down carbohydrate, fat, and protein, respectively.

- Chew your food *very* thoroughly, until it is liquid in your mouth.

- Take betaine hydrochloride (betaine HCl) with each meal; this nutrient helps enhance stomach acidity and speed digestion.

- Avoid eating when stressed; instead, take a few minutes to relax with meditation, deep breathing, or simply being still before sitting down to a meal.

- Don't lie down within three hours of the day's last meal.

- Reduce or eliminate coffee, chocolate, tomatoes, and citrus juices.

- Try an elimination diet.

- Eat more raw fruits and vegetables; these contain enzymes helpful for breaking down food and reducing the time it spends in the stomach.

- Eat cranberries or take cranberry extract; this has been found to reduce the invasion of *H. pylori*.

To Treat Heartburn Naturally:

- Drink fresh juice of potatoes or cabbage (you'll need a vegetable juicer to make this juice), or eat a little raw grated potato.

- Slowly eat a banana, chewing it well.

- Drink some club soda.

- Drink a glass of organic milk or eat a few ounces of plain yogurt.

- Drink a teaspoon of baking soda mixed with 4 to 8 ounces of warm water.

To Prevent Constipation:

- Vegetables, fruit, and whole grains! A diet rich in these foods—especially the first two—will help a great deal with constipation.

- Make sure you're getting 30 or more grams of fiber each day in your food and supplements.

- Repopulate the colon with "good" bacteria—live probiotics, including *L. acidophilus* and *B. bifidus* strains—with each meal or once a day for six weeks.

- Drink eight 8-ounce glasses of water each day.

- Get adequate exercise.

- Go to the toilet whenever the urge strikes; don't hold it for later!

- Reduce stress; if your body is in fight-or-flight mode, your bowel motility is reduced.

To Treat Constipation Naturally:

- Stir 1 teaspoon to 1 tablespoon of psyllium or ground flax into 8 to 12 ounces of water and drink down immediately.

- Take senna or sennoside tablets or cascara sagrada, as directed on package.

- Eat prunes or drink prune juice.

- Take an herbal supplement called *Triphala*, a combination of three Ayurvedic herbs that improves elimination.

- Take 1,000 to 2,000 mg of magnesium oxide before bed.

- Take 5,000 to 10,000 mg of vitamin C; build up gradually to find the right dose.

- If you decide to use an enema, use only saline or water versions, and use them only occasionally—or you can end up making the problem worse.

- Don't strain! Sit down and relax; do some deep breathing; elevate your feet slightly; and let nature take its course.

If the natural remedies you use end up causing diarrhea, be sure to rehydrate and take your supplements on schedule the following day.

THE DIGESTIVE HEALTH SUPPLEMENT PROGRAM

If you are using digestive drugs, take your multivitamin/mineral supplement as recommended in Chapter 2, plus additional supplements to match the doses of the following nutrients.

For replenishing depletions from GI medicines, as well as for improving overall digestive health:

- Calcium: 1,000–1,200 mg as calcium citrate (the most easily absorbed form)

- Folic acid: 400 mcg daily

- Iron: 15 mg, if you are a woman of child-bearing age taking an antacid or H2 blocker

- Magnesium: 400–600 mg daily
- Vitamin B_6: 10–25 mg daily
- Vitamin B_{12}: 200 mcg daily
- Vitamin D: 600–1,000 IU daily
- Zinc: 25–50 mg daily

For increasing low stomach acid:

- Betaine HCl: Follow directions on container; do not use if you have ulcers or are taking drugs that could cause ulcers, including the NSAID drugs, which are covered in Chapter 5
- Digestive enzyme: Take a supplement that contains enzymes that break down protein (proteases), fats (lipases), and milk sugars (lactose), with meals
- Mastic gum: 500 mg, twice daily after meals, for a total of 1,000 mg a day
- Omega-3 fatty acids: 1,000 mg of EPA/DHA from fish oil, twice daily
- Probiotic: High-quality supplement containing 5 billion live bacteria, including *L. acidophilus* and *B. bifidus* strains, twice a day at meals
- Zinc-carnosine: 75 mg twice daily between meals for eight weeks, then 75 mg daily as a maintenance dose

You are what you eat—and absorb. Be sure to eat well, ensure proper digestion, absorption, and elimination. This will go a long way to avoiding chronic problems and dependency on medications, and will promote good health and sustained energy.

SEVEN

Prescriptions for Psychological Health: Antidepressants

We're all prone to mood shifts, and it's only natural to feel blue from time to time. Occasional bouts of sadness may even help us appreciate the good times. In any case, most of us will bounce back within a short time—hours, days, or even a week or two. Others may respond more seriously—withdraw from friends and family, find themselves unable to sleep, and head on a downward spiral toward a severe clinical depression. This affects one in five people at some time in their lives. The symptoms of depression are varied (for a listing, see the inset on page 114), and may occur one at a time or in combination, and generally come upon you gradually. They can be also brought on by a crisis.

As a psychiatrist, I'd like to explain depression and its treatment, both areas badly misunderstood by many patients and their families. At times, even doctors don't have a clear grasp of what depression is and how it is best treated.

Most of us are able to take adversity in stride, yet clearly some people are more resilient than others, depending on genetics, personal history, and lifestyle.

Depression is too often considered to be an issue of "mind over matter." Friends, family, and sadly, even therapists, will tell you that self-discipline is the way you can kick these mind-states. The truth is, rather than being crazy, neurotic, or hopelessly psychologically damaged, you may simply be deficient in certain nutrients. Most mainstream medical practitioners overlook the fact that mood, behavior, and mental performance all depend on your balance of neurotransmitters, the chemical messengers of the brain. It's not just mind over matter, but matter over mind, as well.

The keys to your brain function are the chemical messengers of mind and mood called *neurotransmitters*. As they travel around your brain and nervous system, they help determine how you feel.

Here's the important part: we can influence our brain function by supplying the right nutrients to make our brain cells and neurotransmitters work at their peak.

While there are hundreds of neurotransmitters, the following are the main players:

- *GABA* (gamma-aminobutyric acid) is the "cool" neurotransmitter, relaxing you and calming you down after stress.

- *Epinephrine* (also called adrenaline), made in the adrenal glands, is the "motivator," stimulating you and helping you respond to stress.

- *Dopamine* and *norepinephrine* (also called noradrenaline) are the "feel-good" neurotransmitters, making you feel energized and in control.

> **Symptoms of Depression**
> - Ongoing sad mood
> - Loss of interest or pleasure in activities that the person once enjoyed
> - Significant change in appetite or weight
> - Oversleeping or difficulty sleeping
> - Agitation or unusual slowness
> - Loss of energy
> - Feelings of worthlessness or guilt
> - Difficulty "thinking"—concentrating, making decisions
> - Recurrent thoughts of death or suicide

- *Endorphins* promote that blissful feeling, giving a sense of euphoria.

- *Acetylcholine* works on memory and concentration.

- *Serotonin* is the "happy" and calming neurotransmitter, improving your mood, and helping you to sleep well.

- *Melatonin* helps to keep you in tune with the cycles of nature by responding to seasonal shifts and regulating your inner clock for day and night. It affects your ability to sleep soundly and to dream.

When these neurotransmitters are out of balance, you can feel depressed, anxious, stressed, and unmotivated—or have any other mental problem that you can imagine. On the other hand, with balanced neurotransmitters you are calm, happy, and can think clearly. You are able to handle all the challenges that life throws at you, and enjoy all the wonders as well.

THE FOOD CONNECTION

The protein we eat is broken down by digestive processes into its component amino acids. For brain function, the most important ones are tryptophan, tyrosine, GABA, glutamine, and taurine. They are turned into neurotransmitters with the help of cofactors, or chemical helpers: vitamins B_3 (niacin), B_6 (pyridoxine), folic acid (folate), B_{12} (cyanocobalamin), and C; and the minerals zinc and magnesium. In addition, you need the essential fatty acids that make up about 60 percent of each brain cell. All of these can be supplemented as you'll see later in this chapter.

Then there's glucose required for fuel. Amazingly, this little three-pound organ called the brain can use up to half of the body's glucose (blood sugar) at any one time. That's why we feel so good when we have a sugar hit—it goes right to the brain, which burns it for fuel! The same is true of processed foods, alcohol, and caffeine. You'll get a quick high, but in a short time, it's used up and your body wants more. Stay on that sugar rollercoaster and eventually, you'll start suffering blood sugar swings and increasing mood swings. (See Chapters 2 and 3 for more information on blood-sugar imbalances.)

As I mentioned, you need sufficient amounts of the key neurotransmitters to stay centered, calm, and happy. In depression, there is a lack of mood-stabilizing serotonin and noradrenaline, as well as dopamine, the brain chemicals associated with motivation and pleasure, and derived from tyrosine.

To make serotonin, your brain needs the essential amino acid tryptophan, found in protein-containing foods like turkey, chicken, cottage cheese, avocados, bananas, and wheat germ. Then, eating some carbohydrate along with it helps carry the tryptophan into the brain where it is converted into serotonin. Supplementation with the amino acid 5-hydroxytryptophan (5-HTP) can also help your brain manufacture more serotonin and, unlike tryptophan, it doesn't need carbs for it to get into the brain.

Norepinephrine deficiency often results in cravings for stimulation from sugar, coffee, stress, or alcohol. The amino acids tyrosine and phenylalanine, which can be taken as supplements, convert to dopamine, which helps your brain manufacture more norepinephrine—and the cravings stop!

With anxiety, there is a deficiency in the calming neurotransmitter, GABA, the brain's "antistimulant." Tryptophan-containing foods activate GABA, especially when taken with some carbs, as just mentioned above.

Besides your food intake, there are dozens of reasons why your neurotransmitters may get out of whack, among them: diabetes, liver disease, thyroid imbalance, autoimmune disease, heart disease, high blood pressure, cancer, blood pressure-lowering medications, birth control pills, tranquilizers and stimulants. Depression and anxiety can also be caused by blood sugar imbalances, sex hormone imbalances, food and chemical sensitivities, and toxins, so it might be helpful for you to read about these in my book, *8 Weeks to Vibrant Health* (McGraw-Hill, 2004).

ANTIDEPRESSANTS: WHAT THEY ARE, WHAT THEY DO

Millions of people are taking prescription drugs for depression. Only about half of them find overall relief—besides suffering unpleasant side effects.

My patient Alexandra, mentioned briefly in Chapter 1, is a good case in point. A forty-eight-year-old wife and mother, she came to see me with a variety of health issues: she was taking Prozac, which helped with her depression somewhat, but interfered with her sleeping through the night, so her doctor prescribed another medication for sleep. Alexandra's sex drive was non-existent, likely a side effect of the drug; her hair was falling out in clumps, and she was gaining weight. Her doctor told her that all the symptoms were related to the drug, but he believed it was better than being depressed. She wasn't so sure. When she started having anxiety attacks, he added an anti-anxiety drug, Xanax, which would wear off after an hour or two, and then she'd feel even more anxious. In need of a second opinion, she came to see me.

Since depression, fatigue, and hair loss can be due to low thyroid, I tested her and sure enough, she was *hypothyroid*, or low thyroid. I prescribed thyroid hormone and checked her other hormones, which showed that she was perimenopausal. To help her achieve balance, I prescribed bio-identical hormones, which are female hormones that have the same structure as those made by our bodies. She was also low in vitamins needed to maintain a positive mood—specifically, the B vitamins and vitamin D.

All these plus fish oil, a multivitamin, and some specific amino acids to raise neurotransmitters did the trick. She was able to reduce her dose of antidepressant, and its side effect of anxiety, while still maintaining the antidepressant effect. Then I gradually weaned her off the Xanax and the sleeping medication. A few months later, she was off all the drugs, and happy to report that she was "feeling like (her) old self again."

For most people, the first-line most common treatment for depression is prescription antidepressants. They are among the top-selling drugs in the United States, with 60 million prescriptions per year at a cost of $10 billion. At least 10 percent of adult women and 4 percent of adult men are taking them. They are prescribed for a long list of conditions besides depression, including anxiety, bipolar disorder, chronic pain, eating disorders, and obsessive-compulsive disorder.

While antidepressants may be enormously helpful, even life-saving for some people, they are often overprescribed, at too high a dose, over too long a time, and often before a good medical evaluation has been done.

People are led to believe that the popular selective serotonin reuptake inhibitors and similar antidepressant drugs are totally safe, and that they are repairing an imbalance in their brains. The truth is, these drugs actually *create* an imbalance by altering the action of neurotransmitters, the chemical messengers of the brain. This action has the short-term effect of making the person feel better, but can also have difficult side effects.

CLASSES OF ANTIDEPRESSANT DRUGS

There are several groups of antidepressants, starting with the older tricyclic antidepressants and monoamine oxidase inhibitors (MAOIs) and the newer selective serotonin reuptake inhibitors (SSRIs) and combined serotonin and norepinephrine reuptake inhibitors (SNRIs). There are no known nutrient depletions in the newer antidepressants, although nutrition does have a significant role in treating depression.

TRICYCLIC ANTIDEPRESSANTS: amitriptyline (Elavil), norptriptyline (Aventyl, Pamelor), imipramine (Tofranil), and norimipramine

This older class of antidepressant is used less frequently due to the high number of side effects.

Actions: They work in various ways to affect the actions of norepinephrine and serotonin.

Side effects: These include dizziness, drowsiness, heart palpitations, dry mouth, blurred vision, confusion, weight gain, sweating, rashes, nausea, constipation or diarrhea, difficulty urinating, sexual dysfunction, nightmares, and anxiety.

Nutrients depleted: Vitamin B_2 (riboflavin) and CoQ_{10}.

Needed supplements: Vitamin B_2 (25 mg daily), CoQ_{10} (30–100 mg daily).

MONOAMINE OXIDASE INHIBITORS (MAOIS): isocarboxazid (Marplan), phenelzine (Nardil), and tranylcypromine (Parnate)

These are seldom used, and only when others have failed.

Actions: They work by inhibiting or reducing the levels of the enzyme monoamine oxidase (MAO) that breaks down neurotransmitters in the brain. MAOIs also can cause blood pressure to rise.

Side effects: They can cause dangerously high blood pressure if taken with decongestants, antihistamines, or foods containing tyramine, such as cheese or red wine.

Nutrients depleted: Phenelzine (Nardil) depletes vitamin B_6.

Needed supplements: Vitamin B_6 (25–50 mg daily); sufficient amounts may be part of your multivitamin.

SELECTIVE SEROTONIN REUPTAKE INHIBITORS (SSRIS): citalopram (Celexa, Cipramil, Talohexane), escitalopram (Cipralex, Lexapro), fluoxetine (Fluctin, Fontex, Lovan, Prozac, Sarafem), paroxetine (Aropax, Paxil, Seroxat), and sertraline (Apo-Sertral, Gladem, Lustral, Stimuloton, Serlift, Zoloft)

SSRIs are the most commonly prescribed class of antidepressants.

Action: SSRIs work by tricking the brain into thinking there are more serotonin neurotransmitters than there really are. It does this by stopping the reabsorption of serotonin from the synapse; so, instead of being picked up by the cell and broken down, the serotonin molecule gets to connect with the same receptors several times over. The net effect is an increase of the neurotransmitter's feel-good effects. But you can't fool Mother Nature for very long, as you will see.

Side effects: SSRIs have quite a few side effects, including flattening of emotion; loss of libido and inability to perform sexually or attain orgasm in both men and women; suppressed rapid-eye movement (REM) sleep, the most rejuvenating type of sleep, leading to daytime fatigue; headache; nausea; stomach upset; loss of appetite; and agitation and insomnia. SSRIs may also accelerate bone loss in older people, according to a recent study. New labeling on SSRIs reflect recent findings that in rare cases, SSRIs increase suicidal and violent thinking and behavior.

Nutrients depleted: None reported.

ATYPICAL ANTIDEPRESSANTS: bupropion (Wellbutrin, Zyban), duloxetine (Ariclaim, Cymbalta, Xeristar, Yentreve), venlafaxine (Effexor, Effexor XR)

Atypical antidepressants are a more modern class of antidepressant, used when a patient is more withdrawn due to a lack of norepinephrine (besides being anxious from a lack of serotonin), and needs to have more of the activating neurotransmitters. Often, medications are switched around until the right one is found for the patient.

Action: Atypical antidepressants vary in their effects on reuptake of serotonin, norepinephrine, and dopamine. Bupropion affects norepinephrine and dopamine; duloxetine affects serotonin, norepinephrine, and dopamine; and venlafaxine affects serotonin and norepinephrine. This type of antidepressant medication prevents brain cells from reabsorbing and breaking down the specified chemicals and boosts their levels in the brain.

Side effects: In general, side effects are the same as those of SSRIs plus vivid dreams, increased blood pressure, electric shock sensations (especially when withdrawing), and excessive anxiety, especially at the start of treatment.

Nutrients depleted: None reported.

More Antidepressant Facts You Should Know

Despite the success of antidepressant drugs in treating many people, a study reported in the *New England Journal of Medicine* found that most commonly prescribed antidepressants do not work in at least half of those who take them. You may also have to try one or two or more different antidepressants before you find the one with the greatest benefit and least side effects. If you have been on one of these medications for some time, you may also discover that they can lose effectiveness over time, a condition called *tolerance*. Your doctor may then change the drug, add another one, or increase your dosage.

You must be careful not to stop taking an antidepressant abruptly, which can cause intense withdrawal symptoms. If you do decide to try going off of it, taper gradually with the help of your doctor. Don't substitute the facts from this (or any) book for your doctor's medical opinion. However, you may want to bring up some of this information with your doctor, and follow my suggestions for an easier withdrawal experience.

An excellent resource on the risks, side effects, and withdrawal issues you may encounter when taking antidepressants is Harvard psychiatrist Joseph Glenmullen's *The Antidepressant Solution* (Simon & Schuster, 2000). He warns us that no one really knows the long-term effects of these chemicals on the brain. The book includes convenient symptom lists and graphs that you can fill out during your withdrawal process. I have given these to my own patients to track their progress.

Withdrawal symptoms include agitation, anxiety, hostility, impulsivity, and even suicidal tendencies. I have found that cushioning the withdrawal with specific supplements can ease and shorten the process.

BIPOLAR ILLNESS AND MOOD STABILIZERS

Bipolar disorder is a mood disorder affecting two million Americans. It's not nearly as common as other types of depression. Formerly called "manic-depressive illness," it involves alternating states of depression and mania that follow each other in a cycle, repeatedly. These mood swings may follow each other very closely, within days (rapid cycling); or, the swing from depression to mania or back the other way may be separated by months to years.

CLASSES OF MOOD STABILIZER DRUGS

A variety of medications are used to treat the manic phase, including antidepressants, antipsychotics such as olonzepine (Zyprexa), quetiapine (Seroquel), and haloperidol (Haldol). For more information on antipsychotics, see page 137. Also used are mood stabilizers and anticonvulsants such as valproic acid (Depakote, Depakene), and lamotrigine (Lamictal). They all have a calming effect on the brain, mediated mainly by the neurotransmitter GABA). An older but still reliable drug for bipolar illness is lithium—which we'll cover here, since it's not included in the section on Anticonvulsants in Chapter 8.

MOOD STABILIZER: lithium (Lithobid, Lithonate, Eskalith)

Lithium has long been a mainstay in the treatment of bipolar illness. It is a natural mineral that we require in trace amounts, and is quite low in people with learning disabilities and in violent criminals. While we need a certain amount in order to feel calm, when patients are given too much lithium, they complain about feeling numb, or slowed down, like "in a mental strait-jacket."

Action: Lithium calms the nervous system, likely by its effects on the calming neurotransmitter, GABA.

Side effects: The side effects of lithium can include muscle weakness, fatigue, tremors, loss of appetite, nausea, diarrhea, and thyroid suppression. To avoid toxicity, you need to have your lithium blood levels checked regularly.

Nutrients depleted: Lithium depletes folic acid and inositol. Inositol is a sugar found in cantaloupe, and citrus fruit; it has a calming effect on the mind and body, and I have often successfully prescribed it to bipolar or anxious patients, even those not on lithium.

Needed supplements: Folic acid (400–800 micrograms [mcg] daily), inositol (250–1,000 mg daily in divided doses—for example, 500 mg twice daily).

NUTRIENTS FOR RAISING YOUR MOOD

With the newer antidepressants, drug-induced depletions aren't as much an issue as the nutritional deficiencies that contribute to depression in the first place. On the other hand, we know that certain supplements can greatly *improve* the effect of the drugs described in this chapter. These gentle, safe supplemental nutrients help correct the underlying imbalances, whether or not drugs are part of the picture. Please tell your doctor if you plan on taking them, since they may lower your needed dose of medication.

Amino Acids

Your doctor can actually order a lab test that measures your amino acid levels, so you can precisely target the amino acid supplements that will help you the most. Otherwise, you can figure out which aminos to take based on your symptoms.

Of course, safety, is of utmost importance. Add one amino acid at a time and observe its effects. The only cautions are not to combine the following three mood-enhancing amino acids with MAOIs.

5-HTP (5-hydroxytryptophan)

Derived from tryptophan, 5-HTP is converted into serotonin, causing you to feel relaxed, in a good mood, and able to fall asleep and stay asleep. Another benefit of 5-HTP is that it suppresses appetite. Make sure you are also taking vitamin B_6, which it needs for making serotonin.

Cautions: In rare cases at very high doses, 5-HTP can cause nausea, anxiety, and agitation. For some sensitive individuals it can cause anxiety at normal levels as well. Do not take 5-HTP with SSRIs except under medical guidance. While generally safe to combine, there is a risk of serotonin syndrome—nausea, sweating, headache, and a rise in blood pressure. If that occurs, stop the 5-HTP.

Dose: Take 50–100 mg two to three times daily for daytime usage. To promote sleep, take 50–200 mg one hour before bedtime. Start at the lower dose and gradually increase based on your response.

DL-Phenylalanine and L-Tyrosine

These amino acids can help you get a real boost in mood and energy, relieve pain, and control your appetite. DL-phenylalanine (DLPA) converts to tyrosine, which then is converted to dopamine, norepinephrine, and finally, epinephrine.

Cautions: You could get too much stimulation, causing anxiety, high blood pressure, or insomnia. These shouldn't be taken by people with phenylketonuria or melanomas, or by pregnant or nursing women. Use caution with a history of bipolar illness, because they act as antidepressants and can induce mania.

Dose: Take either 500–1,000 mg of DLPA or tyrosine twice daily on an empty stomach: first thing in the morning then again in mid-afternoon, if needed. Start at the lower dose and gradually increase based on your response. Do not take close to bedtime. Avoid proteins for two hours before or after if possible, since they may interfere with absorption.

B Vitamins

B vitamins are major players in the workings of the nervous system. Most of the B vitamin deficiency diseases strongly affect the mind, mood and memory, as well as energy levels and the ability to handle stress. To curb depression, make sure that your daily intake includes the following dosages of the B vitamins. A high-potency multivitamin may give you most of these dosages; if not, add extra B vitamins as needed.

Vitamin B₁ (Thiamine)

Vitamin B_1 aids in the conversion of sugars into energy. In the brain, glucose is the only source of energy—that's why low blood sugar makes you dizzy and irritable.

Dose: 25 mg daily.

Vitamin B₃ (Niacin)

Extreme vitamin B_3 deficiency, called pellagra, causes psychosis and dementia. Less extreme deficiency can cause milder versions of these mental symptoms. Use non-flush version if desired (see page 70).

Dose: 40–100 mg daily.

Vitamin B₅ (Pantothenic Acid)

Vitamin B_5 is a catalyst, or helper, in making neurotransmitters and "fight or flight" hormones. A deficiency leads to fatigue, depression, and difficulty handling stress.

Dose: 100–500 mg daily.

Vitamin B₆ (Pyridoxine)

Vitamin B_6 is a cofactor in turning the amino acid tryptophan into serotonin. It is depleted by oral contraceptives, and studies show that supplements of B_6 in women taking the pill help to relieve their depression. PMS-related depression similarly has been linked to low B_6 levels, and is relieved by B_6 supplements.

Dose: 20–50 mg daily. Although my usual recommendation for B_6 is 10–25 mg, often with serious depletion you need to take a higher dose. Doses up to 100 mg are quite safe, and I have prescribed even higher doses when needed. Be sure to take it along with other B vitamins to avoid imbalance.

Vitamin B₁₂ (Cyanocobalamin)

Vitamin B_{12} is deficient in 12 to 14 percent of depressed individuals. B_{12}

deficiency is more likely to be a cause of depression in elderly people who don't absorb the nutrient well. In my own clinical experience, elderly individuals that appeared to have Alzheimer's disease have responded remarkably well to a series of B_{12} and folic acid injections, showing an increase in memory, thinking ability, and mood.

Dose: 500–1,000 mcg daily.

Folic Acid/Folate

Folic acid, also known as folate, also helps to prevent depression. Fifteen to thirty-eight percent of adults diagnosed with depressive disorders have been found to have borderline low or deficient blood levels of folic acid. These people are more likely to respond poorly to SSRI therapy, and respond better once folic acid is added.

Dose: 400–800 mcg daily.

Other Nutrients for Boosting Your Mood

SAMe (S-adenosyl methionine)

SAMe (pronounced *sammy*) is a natural mood enhancer made by the body. It is essential in the manufacture of neurotransmitters.

Cautions: High doses may lead to irritability, anxiety, insomnia, or nausea. In people with bipolar disorder, SAMe (like any antidepressant) may trigger a manic episode, so they should be monitored carefully.

Dose: Take 200 mg of SAMe once or twice daily, between meals, increasing gradually to a maximum of 1,600 mg a day, if needed. Generally, 400–800 mg a day will do.

Omega-3 Fatty Acids

The omega-3 fatty acids are important not just for health; they're important for happiness, too. The omega-3 fatty acids EPA and DHA are found in high concentrations in fatty, carnivorous fish such as herring, mackerel, tuna, and salmon. (Smaller amounts are found in other fish.) In countries where more fish is consumed, there is a lower rate of depression. Omega-3 fish oils can elevate your mood. Besides their use for depression, studies have shown that fish oil is helpful for bipolar disorder, as well. To ensure that you get enough of the essential omega-3s, eat fish (salmon, sardines, tuna, mackerel, cod) two to three times a week. For more information on the use of omega-3 fatty acids in depression, read *The Omega-3 Connection: The Groundbreaking Antidepression Diet and Brain Program* by Andrew Stoll, M.D. (Free Press, 2002),

Caution: Be careful about the source and potential contamination level of the fish you're choosing. Oceans Alive (www.oceansalive.org) has a great reference list you can consult to stay up-to-date whenever you shop for fish.

Dose: For depression, take 1,000–2,000 mg EPA plus DHA daily (if you are vegetarian, take one tablespoon of flaxseed oil instead); for bipolar illness, try 8 grams (8,000 mg) or so a day.

While research has used 10 grams to successfully treat bipolar disorder, I have found that if omega-3 fish oil is combined with other supplements in this chapter they work together, and the required dose is more like 4–6 grams (4,000–6,000 mg). Note: To take this high a dose of EPA/DHA without swallowing a dozen capsules a day, you will need to use a highly concentrated fish oil supplement that's 90 percent composed of these fatty acids.

Vitamin D

Vitamin D is a fat-soluble vitamin that's made in the skin during exposure to sunlight. It's also abundant in liver, fish liver oils, and fortified dairy products, egg yolks, salmon, sardines, cream, butter, and liver. Symptoms of vitamin D deficiency include unexplained weakness, pain in the joints, and depression, especially seasonal affective disorder (SAD). If you avoid sun in the summer, take it all year round. Vitamin D is fat-soluble, meaning that it can be stored up in the body, and that it can accumulate to toxic levels if you take too much. You can have your doctor test your vitamin D levels in the form of *25-hydroxy-vitamin D.*

Dose: 1,000 (international units) IU a day throughout the winter.

Saint John's Wort (*Hypericum perforatum*)

Dozens of studies have proved Saint John's wort's ability to relieve mild to moderate depression. It's been shown to be effective in 60 to 80 percent of people who take it. It compares well with the prescription antidepressants but without their side effects. It likely enhances serotonin, like the SSRI antidepressants, as well as dopamine and norepinephrine.

Cautions: It may cause allergic reactions, rashes, gastrointestinal upset, or sun sensitivity in some people. It can cause anxiety or insomnia if taken too close to bedtime. It can reduce the potency of digoxin (a heart medication, see Chapter 8), protease inhibitors (taken as treatment for AIDS, see Chapter 8) or cyclosporin (an immunosuppressant taken by organ transplant patients), or even birth control pills (see also, Chapter 8). Not recommended for use during pregnancy or nursing. If combined with an SSRI or 5-HTP, there's the (very slight) possibility of serotonin syndrome—headache, an increase in body temperature, and heavy sweating. Stop the St. John's wort and seek medical help if this occurs.

Dose: Start with one or two capsules of 300 mg of an extract with 0.3 percent *hypericin*, starting in the morning with breakfast. If it doesn't have a noticeable effect in a week, add another capsule at lunchtime, for a total of 900 mg daily. You can also take your entire dose in the morning, because the herb is quite long acting.

Rhodiola (*Rhodiola rosea*)

Rhodiola is an adaptogenic herb, meaning that it helps to regulate your system in response to stress. Russian research shows that rhodiola can enhance your body's production of serotonin, dopamine, and norepinephrine, enabling it to both lift your mood and calm your nerves. For more information, see *The Rhodiola Revolution* (Rodale Press, 2004).

Cautions: Since it is energizing, it may trigger a manic episode in those with bipolar disorder.

Dose: Use 100–300 mg of a product standardized to 3 percent *rosavins* and 0.8 to 1.0 percent *salidrosides.*

More Helpful Mood Enhancers

- Calcium: Low levels of calcium cause nervousness, irritability, and numbness. **Dose:** 1,000 mg daily.

- Iron: In premenopausal women, depression may be a symptom of chronic iron deficiency anemia. **Dose:** Up to 15 mg daily.

- Magnesium: Deficiency in this mineral can result in depression, confusion, and anxiety. **Dose:** 250–500 mg daily.

- Vitamin C: Deficiencies in vitamin C can lead to depression. Stress, pregnancy, nursing, surgery, inflammatory disease, and infection will all deplete your vitamin C supply. So will aspirin, tetracycline, and birth control pills. **Dose: 250–1,000 mg twice daily** (it doesn't last long in the body, so it's best to take it twice).

- Zinc: Low levels can cause apathy, lack of appetite, and fatigue. **Dose: 15–30 mg daily.**

OTHER SELF-CARE THERAPIES

There are various types of psychotherapy or "talk" therapy, which can be very helpful in dealing with depression. Some of the more rapid therapies are EMDR (Eye Movement Desensitization and Reprocessing, EMDR.com); guided imagery; EFT (Emotional Freedom Techniques, emofree.org); and Voice Dialogue, developed by Drs. Hal and Sidra Stone (www.delos-inc.com). There are also useful self-regulation techniques such as meditation. Any form of therapy works much better once your brain chemistry is balanced, whether by medication, diet, or supplements.

A SUPPLEMENT PROGRAM FOR PSYCHOLOGICAL HEALTH

In conclusion, a healthy diet, exercise, a positive attitude, and the appropriate supplements can boost your mood quite well, with or without the use of medication. If you are taking medication, be sure to supplement with the cofactors that make neurotransmitters, especially the B vitamins. By combining medication with nutrients, you will most likely cut down the dose needed, and so have fewer and milder side effects, and an overall better quality of life.

For depletions:

- If taking tricyclics, take 25 mg B_2 and 30–100 mg CoQ_{10}.

- If taking the MAOI phenelzine (Nardil), take 25–50 mg B_6.

- If taking lithium, take 400–800 mcg folic acid and 250–1,000 mg inositol in divided doses.

For general nutritional balance for good mental health:

- B vitamins (these doses may be found in a high-dose multivitamin; add extra amounts as needed)
  - B_1 25 mg daily

- ○ B_2 40–100 mg daily
- ○ B_5 100–500 mg daily
- ○ B_6 20–50 mg daily
- ○ B_{12} 500–1,000 mcg daily
- ○ Folic acid 400–800 mcg daily
- Omega-3 fatty acids: 1,000–2,000 mg of EPA/DHA from fish oil daily
- Vitamin D: 1,000 IU daily, especially in winter

For creating neurotransmitter balance in depression:

- B vitamins: (see above)
- Calcium: 1,000 mg daily
- 5-HTP: 50–200 mg daily
- Iron: 15 mg for women of child-bearing age
- Magnesium: 250–500 mg daily
- Phenylalanine and/or tyrosine: 500–1,000 mg twice daily
- SAMe: 400–800 mg daily
- Vitamin C: 250–1,000 mg twice daily
- Zinc: 15–30 mg daily

For relieving depressive symptoms:

- Rhodiola: 100–300 mg daily
- St. John's wort: 900 mg of an extract with 0.3 percent *hypericin*

For bipolar disorder:

- B vitamins: (see above)
- Calcium: 1,000 mg daily
- Iron: 15 mg for women of child-bearing age
- Omega-3 fatty acids: 5,000–10,000 mg of EPA/DHA from fish oil daily
- Magnesium: 250–500 mg daily
- Vitamin C: 250–1,000 mg twice daily
- Zinc: 15–30 mg daily

EIGHT

Prescriptions for Other Conditions:
Antibiotics and Drugs for Birth Control, Bipolar Disorder, Cancer, and More

A side from the drugs we've covered in previous chapters, there are countless others you or a loved one may find you need to get through a health crisis. Other drugs are necessary for the management of chronic, possibly life-altering or life-threatening diseases. Some of these diseases respond well to natural therapies; others can only be managed with medications. No matter what condition you find yourself wrestling with, know that excellent nutrition and specific supplementation will help any person, ill or well, to get the most out of life. This is especially true when powerful, depleting medicines are needed.

Certain drugs are a fact of life for people who are severely ill with diseases like AIDS, rheumatoid arthritis, tuberculosis, heart rhythm irregularities (*arrhythmias*) or inflammatory bowel diseases such as Crohn's disease. Other medicines are needed by people with chronic conditions such as epilepsy, schizophrenia, or Parkinson's disease. Oral contraceptives or estrogen replacement therapy may be a necessary part of pregnancy prevention or dealing with menopause. Cancer chemotherapy is a grim, but potentially life-saving, reality for some. And even healthy people sometimes come down with infections that require antibiotic treatment.

This chapter will give you an overview of the depletions you can expect with these medications and how to supplement them. Many of the dosages can be found in a high-potency daily multivitamin; if the dosage of one or more nutrients falls short of these recommendations, you can add more of individual nutrients as needed. I'll cover these drugs in alphabetical order, mostly by their drug class or indication, with a few individual drugs in each class.

- AIDS medications

- Antibiotics

- Anticonvulsants (used to treat epilepsy and bipolar disorder)
- Anti-obesity drugs
- Antipsychotics (used to treat schizophrenia, bipolar disorder, and severe pain)
- Barbiturates and benzodiazepines (sedatives)
- Cancer chemotherapy
- Colchicine (for gout)
- Corticosteroids (used to treat inflammatory conditions like rheumatoid arthritis, severe asthma, and inflammatory bowel disease; also used to slow cancer growth)
- Digoxin (for heart arrhythmia)
- Isoniazid (for tuberculosis)
- Levodopa/carbidopa (for Parkinson's disease)
- Methotrexate (for rheumatoid arthritis and cancer chemotherapy)
- Oral contraceptives/estrogens (for birth control, menstrual regulation, or menopausal symptoms)
- Osteoporosis drugs
- Sulfasalazine (for rheumatoid arthritis)

AIDS MEDICATIONS

At this writing, over twenty AIDS/HIV medications are available. They are usually used in combinations called *antiretroviral cocktails*. They block most of the stages of viral replication, prolonging the lives of people with AIDS/HIV dramatically.

The drugs most commonly used to treat human immunodeficiency virus (HIV, the virus that causes AIDS) and acquired immunodeficiency syndrome (AIDS, the immune system disorder) fall into two categories: *non-nucleoside reverse transcriptase inhibitors* and *nucleoside reverse transcriptase inhibitors*. Zidovudine, or AZT, is the best known. Both AIDS and the medicines used to treat it can cause loss of appetite, mouth sores, diarrhea, and nausea, and can interfere with good nutrition. People who live with HIV/AIDS have to be extremely careful to avoid food-borne "bugs" that a healthy immune system could handle, but that their reduced defenses can't stamp out.

Action: The HIV virus destroys cells that belong to the immune system. Both classes of drugs inhibit *reverse transcriptase*, the enzyme that HIV needs in order to replicate itself.

Side effects: These vary from drug to drug, and may include headache, nausea, muscle pain, dizziness, diarrhea, anemia, rash, peripheral neuropathy (burning, stinging, stiffness, tickling, or numbness in feet, toes, or hands), hair loss, weight loss, or menstrual problems.

Nutrients depleted: Carnitine, copper, vitamin B_{12}, and zinc.

Needed supplements:

- **L-carnitine:** 500–2,000 milligrams (mg) of L-carnitine daily in divided doses. A special esterified form called acetyl-L-carnitine (at the same dosage) is preferable when the brain and nervous system are involved.

  Carnitine is an amino acid produced in the body from an essential amino acid called lysine. It's highly concentrated in muscle, heart, liver, and kidneys, and is important for regulating heart function. Carnitine also transports fats into cells to be burned for energy in the mitochondria. Deficiency symptoms include elevated blood fats (such as cholesterol and triglycerides), lack of energy, muscle weakness, and blood sugar imbalances.

  Athletes often use carnitine supplements to enhance energy and endurance, while others use it as a weight-loss supplement. In HIV/AIDS, supplemental carnitine may be used to raise its levels in the cells; research suggests that this really helps to control nerve damage, which is a common consequence of HIV/AIDS and its treatment with drugs. (Carnitine is also useful for diabetic neuropathy, another kind of nerve damage.) Other benefits include prevention of muscle and fat wasting, and reduced levels of "bad" LDL cholesterol and triglycerides.

  Studies show that carnitine may help to slow the progression of Alzheimer's disease and heart failure. It's also a promising therapy for *angina* (chest pain from poor blood flow to the heart muscle) and *intermittent claudication* (pain in the lower legs caused by poor circulation, generally due to *arteriosclerosis*, or hardening of the arteries).

  The best food sources of carnitine are red meats like steak and ground beef, but even those sources offer only about 80 mg per serving—far less than the amount recommended as a supplement.

  Carnitine at high doses (more than 2 grams or 2,000 mg a day) can reduce thyroid hormone activity or the effectiveness of thyroid hormone replacement.

- **Copper:** 2–3 mg per day—a dose you should be able to get from your multivitamin. Copper is a component of hemoglobin, the protein that carries oxygen in the red blood cells. It also acts as a coenzyme in several of the body's significant biochemical reactions, and is important for cardiovascular health. Deficiency symptoms include loss of color in hair and skin; low body temperature; fatigue; anemia; and lowered immune resistance to infection. High-dose zinc (much higher than 25 mg per day) can deplete copper.

- **Vitamin B$_{12}$:** 500–2,000 mcg per day. Deficiency exists in about a third of people with AIDS. If you are having digestive issues, choose a sublingual B$_{12}$ supplement or talk to your doctor about B$_{12}$ injections. Supplements of B$_{12}$ may inhibit viral invasion into certain types of immune cells. Added bonus: supplements of B$_{12}$ may inhibit viral invasion into certain types of immune cells.

- **Zinc:** 25–100 mg per day.

ANTIBIOTICS

Let's say you go to the doctor with a bad cold or a case of bronchitis, which is almost always caused by a virus. The doctor tells you that no drug can get rid of what you already have, but he may then write you a prescription for an antibiotic—"to prevent secondary infection," he says. Relieved that there is *something* you can take, you go fill your script and dutifully take your medication for ten days . . . for an infection that would have gone away by itself, and that the antibiotic probably did nothing to help.

In the process, you've depleted your body of several important nutrients—especially the "good" probiotic bacteria that help maintain immunity and gastrointestinal health. And you may have contributed in a small way to the growing problem of antibiotic resistance. As antibiotics are used more and more often, bacterial strains that are resistant to those drugs evolve and spread. As a result, the drugs we've come to count on to get rid of truly dangerous infections don't work nearly as well as they used to.

When do you really need an antibiotic? That's a conversation for you to have with your doctor. If you are being evaluated for some sort of infectious condition, ask whether it is likely to be viral; if he isn't sure, you can ask for a culture to be performed. Ask whether your condition is likely to resolve on its own, and whether you can try medicines to relieve pain or sleeplessness—such as decongestants or acetamino-phen—while allowing your immune system to do its best to knock out the bug that's infected you. You can always take your antibiotic prescription home and fill it later if you start to feel worse.

Remember that symptoms of acute inflammation, like fever, runny nose, cough, and body aches, are signs that your immune system is doing its job. Your body is trying to "burn up" and dispose of the infection. Suppressing the infection with antibiotics interferes with the immune system's job—and it needs to be run through its paces every so often to stay in shape. When you "come down with something," see it as an opportunity for your body to clean house and come out the other side renewed.

Instead of running to the doc for an antibiotic, support your body. Bundle up and stay warm; rest; drink lots of fluids; eat little to no food, depending on your appetite. Avoid sugar, which lowers immunity dramatically. Use immune-supporting herbs and nutrients like echinacea, astragalus, and vitamin C (try 1,000 mg every couple of hours).

One of the best books on natural ways to support immunity is *Immunotics* by Robert Rountree, M.D., and Carol Colman (Perigee Trade, 2001). It addresses not only ways to boost an underactive immune system, but also ways to temper an overreacting immune system—the cause of allergy and inflammatory disease.

Action: Each antibiotic works through a slightly different mechanism to kill or disable bacteria without damaging healthy body cells. Some antibiotics hamper the bacteria's ability to build cell walls; some prevent bacteria from reproducing their genetic material; and so on. Some antibiotics can kill many different types of bacteria, while others are highly specific to one or a few types.

Side effects: Upset stomach, diarrhea, vaginal yeast infections; rarely, colitis caused by *Clostridium difficile* bacteria.

Nutrients depleted: Biotin, inositol, vitamins B_1 (thiamine), B_2 (riboflavin), B_3 (niacin) B_5 (pantothenic acid), B_6 (pyridoxine) B_{12} (cyanocobalamin), vitamin K, and probiotics. Additionally, fluoroquinolones (any antibiotic that has a generic name that ends with the suffix "-floxacin," including the well-known ciprofloxacin, brand name Cipro) deplete calcium and iron; tetracyclines (end with suffix "-cycline") deplete calcium and magnesium; trimethoprim-containing antibiotics (brand names Trimpex, Proloprim, or Primsol) deplete folic acid; and penicillins (end with suffix "-cillin") deplete potassium.

Needed supplements: The doses of magnesium, iron, calcium, and potassium contained in a good multivitamin (see Chapter 2) should cover your needs for these nutrients during a course of antibiotic therapy. You may need to restore other nutrients depleted with the following additional supplements:

- **B-complex vitamins:** supplement with a B complex or multivitamin that contains 25 mg of B_1, 25 mg of B_2, 50 mg of B_3, 50 mg of B_6, 400–800 micrograms (mcg) of folic acid, 10 mcg of B_{12}, and 50 mg each of biotin and B_5 (pantothenic acid).

- **Inositol:** 100–1,000 mg per day is adequate. (The RDA is 100 mg per day.) Inositol is part of the B-vitamin complex, and is likely to be included in a B-vitamin or multivitamin formulation. For more information, see lithium under Mood Stabilizer Drugs on page 120.

- **Probiotics:** Choose a supplement that contains at least one billion live organisms per daily dose. Antibiotics kill "good" bacteria, including *Lactobacillus acidophilus* (*L. acidophilus*) and *Bifidobacterium bifidum* (*B. bifidum*). These are *probiotics,* or bacteria that normally live in and on the human body, concentrated mostly in the digestive and genital/urinary systems. They get a place to live; in return, we get their help keeping yeasts and less friendly bacteria at bay, and in maintaining optimal digestive health.

  Probiotic bacteria have been used to make cultured foods like sourdough bread, miso, sauerkraut, and yogurt for thousands of years. Societies that eat a lot of cultured foods tend to be longer lived and healthier. Probiotics have also been found to help relieve the diarrhea that may be caused by antibiotics. Yeast overgrowth is a side effect of antibiotic therapy, which is why women often get yeast infection following a course of antibiotics. Probiotics *competitively inhibit* yeast growth—that is, they compete for space and resources.

  Yeasts aren't killed by antibiotics, but probiotics are. Supplementing with probiotics should help prevent yeast overgrowth when used along with antibiotics. Continue to supplement for at least two weeks after finishing the medication.

  While taking an antibiotic, also eat yogurt (plain, live-culture, organic) and other cultured foods regularly. Take your probiotic supplement as far as possible in time from your medication. Aside from *L. acidophilus* and *B. bifidum*, you may find that your supplement contains one or more of the following bacteria, which have all been studied and found to benefit health: *L. bulgaricus, L. casei, L. gasseri, L. plantarum, B. lactis, B. longum, Enterococcus faecium,* and *Saccharomyces boulardii* (a friendly yeast).

- **Vitamin K:** 30–100 mcg per day. Vitamin K is required for proper blood clotting. It is normally made by intestinal bacteria, but those good bugs are killed off by antibiotic therapy. Deficiency is rare, but when it occurs, life-threatening bleeding can result from the smallest injury. Vitamin K may also play a part in bone health and osteoporosis prevention. Your multivitamin should provide 30–100 mcg, which is an adequate dose.

ANTICONVULSANTS/MOOD STABILIZERS

These medicines, which are the fifth top-selling group of drugs in the United States, affect brain chemistry in ways that prevent seizures. They stabilize mood, and are used to treat bipolar disorder. They're also used for pain reduction when nothing else works, and to prevent migraine headaches. (Hint for migraines: try magnesium, 400–500 mg daily, which has actually stopped chronic migraines in a number of my patients.)

There are several classes of anticonvulsant drugs, and only a few are known to cause nutrient depletion: phenytoin (Dilantin), carbamazepine (Tegretol, Carbatrol, Epitrol), primidone (Mysoline), methsuxamide (Celontin), valproic acid (Depakote, Depacon, Depakene), topiramate (Topomax) and gabapentin (Neurontin). Restoring depleted nutrients is particularly important when medications are needed long-term, as these often are.

Action: Anticonvulsants have various modes of action. People with epilepsy may need to use more than one drug at the same time to control seizures.

Side effects: As a class of medications, they have significant side effects, including dizziness, drowsiness, fatigue, headache, confusion, skin rash, abdominal pain, nausea, vomiting, lack of appetite, swollen feet, and weight gain or weight loss. Anticonvulsants are a problem in pregnancy since they are known to cause major birth defects. Some evidence suggests that anticonvulsants may raise risk of suicide or suicidal thinking. Stopping these medicines suddenly can cause withdrawal symptoms that include anxiety, nausea, pain, sweating, and insomnia—and seizures.

Nutrients depleted: The drug phenytoin depletes biotin, calcium, folic acid, and vitamins D and K, plus vitamins B_1 and B_{12}; primidone depletes biotin and folic acid; and valproic acid depletes carnitine. Note: If you're taking primidone or carbamazepine, note that vitamin B_3 interferes with the breakdown of the drugs, and can cause an unsafely high drug level.

Needed supplements: Depending on the drug you are using, you'll use:

- **Calcium:** 1,000–1,200 mg daily with 400–600 mg of magnesium.

- **Carnitine:** 500–2,000 mg daily of L-carnitine or acetyl-L-carnitine.

- **Vitamin B-complex:** Use a B-complex or multivitamin that contains 25 mg of B_1, 25 mg of B_2, 50 mg of B_3, 50 mg of B_6, 400–800 mcg of folic acid, 10 mcg of B_{12}, and 50 mg each of biotin and B_5.

- **Vitamin D:** 1,000 international units (IU) daily.

- **Vitamin K:** Obtain 30–100 mcg of this vitamin through your multivitamin supplement.

ANTI-OBESITY DRUGS

The first thing I'll tell you about these drugs is that they don't work very well. Sure, they might help you lose a little bit of extra weight, but they only help for as long as you use (or tolerate) them. They don't, in any truly significant way, help people who need it the most—people who are obese and suffer health risks because of this.

The latest weight-loss wonder, over-the-counter (OTC) orlistat (Alli), promises that "if you could lose 10 pounds through dieting, you could lose 15 pounds with hard work and Alli." Orlistat is also available by prescription as the brand-name product Xenical. Since the drug's actions rely on binding 25 percent of the fats you consume in your gut and passing them through your body unabsorbed, there's no focus on the *real* reason that most people get fat: *too much refined carbohydrate.* No wonder the drugs don't have much effect.

Action: Orlistat prevents the digestion and absorption of fat in the intestine by blocking the action of lipase, an enzyme that helps break down fat.

Side effects: The drug's side effects are more likely if you go off the wagon and eat a meal with a bit more fat in it. In this situation, you're at substantial risk for gas, "oily spotting," loose stools, and possible partial loss of bowel control. In other words, you may poop in your pants. Who needs it?

Nutrients depleted: If you do decide you want to try Xenical or Alli's program—which, like most weight-loss regimens, involves drastic dietary changes and exercise—you can also expect to be depleted of important fatty acids and fat-soluble nutrients, including vitamins A, D, E, K, and the carotenes.

Needed supplements:

- **High-potency multivitamin:** Use a multivitamin that contains all of the fat-soluble nutrients and with a meal for better absorption.
- **Omega-3 fish oils:** It may be beneficial to take fish oil supplements between doses of orlistat to replenish your body's levels of omega-3 fats; use a supplement that delivers 1,000–3,000 mg of combined DHA/EPA.

ANTIPSYCHOTICS

Drugs in this class are mostly prescribed to people who have schizophrenia, bipolar disorder, or other mental illnesses that involve breaks from reality. They are sometimes prescribed off-label—without FDA approval—for anxiety disorders, post-traumatic stress disorder (PTSD), insomnia, and for Tourette's syndrome (where the person has "tics," involuntary movements and uncontrollable vocal sounds). These drugs are sometimes referred to as *neuroleptics*, a term that means "to take hold of one's nerves."

Typical antipsychotics are a class of older drugs that includes chlorpromazine (Ormazine, Thorazine), fluphenazine (Permitil, Prolixin), haloperidol (Haldol), and thioridazine (Mellaril).

Atypical antipsychotics are a newer subclass that includes aripiprazole (Abilify), olanzapine (Zyprexa), paliperidone (INVEGA, Simap), quetiapine (Seroquel), risperidone (Risperdal), and ziprasidone (Geodon, Zeldox).

Action: These drugs reduce psychotic symptoms by affecting dopamine activity in the brain.

Side effects: Side effects of typical antipsychotics include anxiety, agitation, irregular heartbeat, blurred vision, intense restlessness (*akathisia*), stiff movements (Parkinson's-like symptoms), or painful muscle spasms. Over time, *tardive dyskinesia* can develop; this side effect causes repetitive, uncontrolled movements, such as grimacing; smacking, puckering and pursing of the lips; and rapid eye blinking. Atypical antipsychotics are somewhat less likely to have these side effects, but they can occur. The atypicals can cause substantial weight gain, disruptions in blood sugar control, and even diabetes.

Nutrients depleted: Chlorpromazine, fluphenazine, and thiorizadine deplete CoQ_{10}, melatonin, and vitamin B_2; haloperidol depletes CoQ_{10}. Although there's not as much information on depletions with the newer atypical medicines, their mode of action and side-effect profiles are similar enough to expect that they will deplete the same nutrients as the older, typical antipsychotics.

Needed supplements:

- **CoQ_{10}:** 30–100 mg daily. Choose a version that's packaged with oil for better absorption, take it with your omega-3 oil supplement, or sprinkle powdered CoQ_{10} on a food that contains fat, such as nut butter or buttered toast.

- **Manganese (optional):** 25 mg daily. Evidence from studies conducted by San Francisco-based psychiatrist Richard Kunin show that supplementing with manganese can often help treat tardive dyskinesia (TD). Based on these findings, it's sensible for anyone on antipsychotics to take 25 mg per day for prevention. Higher doses up to 60 mg per day may reverse existing TD. High-dose vitamin E (800–1,600 IU) may also aid in TD prevention, based on a large study by renowned psychiatrist David Hawkins.

- **Melatonin:** 3 mg at bedtime. Melatonin is a hormone made at nightfall. It's built out of the neurotransmitter serotonin, in a small gland in the brain called the pineal gland. This hormone is also a powerful antioxidant. It can be used in low doses (up to 3 mg) as a supplement to aid in deeper sleep or to naturally treat insomnia or jet lag.

  Melatonin is another option for preventing and treating tardive dyskinesia. In a double-blind trial, 10 mg of melatonin each night for six weeks in patients with TD reduced abnormal movements by 23.8 percent. Similar changes were seen in only 8.4 percent of the placebo (dummy pill) group.

  For more information on natural approaches to mental illness, see alternativementalhealth.com, www.nutritional-healing.com.au, and other resources in the back of the book.

- **Vitamin B_2:** 25–100 mg daily.

BARBITURATES AND BENZODIAZEPINES

The first of the barbiturates was developed in the early 1900s, and by the 1950s it was obvious that there was a substantial risk of addiction and dependency in people who took them. They're tranquilizers, primarily used now to treat epilepsy (in combination with anticonvulsants) and as anesthetics.

In common practice, these drugs—such as phenobarbital, secobarbital (Seconal), and amobarbital (Amytal)—are too risky to use for anxiety disorders, and have been replaced by the benzodiazepines.

Diazepam (Valium) was the little yellow benzodiazepine pill made famous by the Rolling Stones' song "Mother's Little Helper." Other benzodiazepines include alprazolam (Xanax), bromazepam (Lexomil), lorazepam (Ativan), clonazepam (Klonopin), temazepam (Restoril), chlordiazepoxide (Librium), flurazepam (Dalmane), and triazolam (Halcion). They all work by increasing activity of the calming neurotransmitter, GABA.

Action: Barbiturates and benzodiazepines both work by affecting the activity of *gamma-aminobutyric acid* (GABA), a neurotransmitter with soothing, relaxant effects. If you do have to take a barbiturate, be aware that it depletes a few nutrients.

Side effects: Benzodiazepines are meant to be prescribed only for short periods of time (two to three weeks). Over longer periods they produce *tolerance*, or the need for more to get the same effect, and *addiction*, with severe withdrawal symptoms. Other side effects include dulled awareness and brain function. Even the day after taking one at bedtime, serious accidents aren't uncommon. Sudden withdrawal can lead to intense anxiety, insomnia, tremors, mental impairment, seizures and even, death. They must be withdrawn slowly under medical supervision.

Nutrients depleted: Barbiturates deplete biotin, folic acid, and vitamins D and K. Benzodiazepines deplete these nutrients, plus calcium and melatonin.

Needed supplements (benzodiazepines and barbiturates):

- **Calcium:** 1,000–1,200 mg daily with 400–600 mg of magnesium.
- **Folic acid:** 400–800 mcg daily.
- **Vitamin D:** 1,000 IU daily.
- **Vitamin K:** 30–100 mcg daily.

Instead of the benzodiazepines and barbiturates, I prescribe the following calming supplements to my patients. They can be used singly, or combined in existing off-the-shelf formulas:

- **5-HTP:** 100–200 mg at bedtime

- **GABA:** 500 mg at bedtime

- **L-theanine:** 200 mg, one to three times daily as needed

- **Melatonin:** 0.5–3 mg at bedtime

- **Valerian:** 200–600 mg at bedtime

I have prescribed these in various combinations for my patients who were withdrawing from benzodiazepines or the newer sleeping pills such as Ambien (zolpidem). As far as Ambien goes: despite claims of Ambien's being "not quite a benzodiazepine" and non-addictive, this has not been so in the many cases I've seen.

Benzodiazepines (and Ambien) must be withdrawn very slowly under close medical supervision, sometimes over several months. Stopping these drugs suddenly can bring on seizures, severe anxiety, insomnia, nightmares, abdominal pain, palpitations, loss of balance, sweating and quite a long list of other symptoms.

CANCER CHEMOTHERAPY

Chemotherapy. Just the word is enough to bring up a wave of anxiety. When we think of chemo, we think of hair loss, vomiting, nausea, and an overall inability to keep up with the demands of life. While chemo is often a hard road, nutritional and dietary changes can reduce the side effects of this difficult medical treatment.

Action: Many drugs belong in this category. Most work to interfere with the replication of cancer cells, though they also destroy normal cells in the process.

Side effects: These vary, depending on the drug; most commonly they include nausea, vomiting, diarrhea, fatigue, anemia, mouth sores, hair loss, changes in taste and smell, infertility, early menopause, fatigue, pain in hands and feet due to nerve damage, bone loss, excess tear production, and memory loss.

Nutrients depleted: Cancer chemotherapy can cause nausea, loss of appetite, and vomiting, all of which have dramatic impact on nutritional status. All chemo drugs act on rapidly dividing cells (including tumors, the lining of the mouth and the rest of the GI tract, and hair follicles), which impacts the body's ability to absorb nutrients from foods. It can bring on intestinal inflammation and destroy the tiny *villi* that line the small intestines and absorb nutrients into the bloodstream. This can make eating painful and may cause diarrhea.

Individual chemotherapy drugs have different potential for GI side effects, and this is a topic for you and your oncology team to discuss. Any way you slice it, chemotherapy drugs have the potential to impose drastic depletions in every class of nutrient, including proteins, fats, and micronutrients (vitamins and minerals). Some pointers:

- *Eat healthfully.* Do what you can to eat a very healthy diet while undergoing chemo. This is probably the most important step you can take towards helping yourself to heal. By supporting your internal environment, you can amp up your body's ability to resist the cancer. Ever notice, in the forest, that parasitic fungi don't grow on all trees? They like to grow on trees that aren't in good health. The same goes for cancers and most other kinds of illness.

- *Say no to sugars and yes to whole plant foods.* Strictly limit sugars and eat lots of vegetables and fruit.

- *Consider a macrobiotic diet.* Some cancer patients find that a macrobiotic diet—which consists of cooked whole grains, vegetables, beans, seaweed, and small amounts of fish—is easier to stomach than a standard diet when undergoing cancer treatment. This may sound foreign to you, but when faced with the serious malnutrition that often accompanies cancer, you may find this a real boon, as others have. For more information, see Michio Kushi's books: *The Cancer Prevention Diet* (St. Martins Griffin, 1994) and *The Macrobiotic Way* (Avery, 2004).

- *Multivitamin.* Take a high-potency, iron-free multivitamin that supplies your body with plenty of antioxidants (vitamins A, C, E, and selenium). Work with your medical team to find a multivitamin that you can keep down—this may mean using a liquid or chewable version. Take your multi with food to aid absorption.

- *Glutamine.* Take 500 mg three times daily. Protect your GI tract by taking L-glutamine, an amino acid that is the intestinal tract's favorite fuel source. It has proven benefit in reducing GI inflammation and nausea.

- *Flaxseeds.* Ground flaxseeds help to create a protective barrier along the intestinal walls; stir a tablespoon or two into oatmeal or cooked whole grains.

- *Milk thistle, an herb with a long history of use as a liver tonic,* is helpful in supporting the liver, your body's 'detox factory'—which is dealing with a high load of chemicals as you undergo chemotherapy. Take 240 mg two to three times daily. Use a milk thistle extract (which is made from the plant's seed) that contains 80% *silymarin,* the herb's active ingredient.

- *Lots of water.* Drink eight to ten glasses of water daily.

- *Vitamin K,* a nutrient essential for blood clotting, is depleted by most chemo drugs. Talk with your oncologist about supplementing 500–1,000 mcg per day to help prevent bruising and bleeding.

- *Omega-3 fatty acids* (1,000–3,000 mg of combined EPA and DHA per day) may help chemo be more effective, while helping to prevent extreme loss of muscle mass known as *cachexia.*

- *Medicinal mushrooms.* Cancer patients may also wish to investigate medicinal mushrooms (such types as reishi, shiitake, cordyceps, maitake, agaracus, and coriolus) as immune-boosting companions to chemotherapy. These medicinal mushrooms are sources of anti-tumor and immunity-modulating polysaccharides (a type of carbo-hydrate) that have been extensively researched. Formulas containing concentrated extracts of medicinal mushrooms are available; talk with your oncologist about which he or she might recommend.

- *Acupuncture and traditional Chinese medicine (TCM).* Many cancer patients also turn to acupuncture and TCM to help them get through the rigors of chemo.

- *Use herbs if you need help relaxing.* Support your program by getting plenty of sleep and taking steps to cope with stress. For better sleep and relaxation, it's safe to use herbs such as valerian (150–300 mg) and passionflower (300–450 mg).

  Note: Avoid St. John's wort while undergoing chemo, as it has been found to interfere with the action of some chemo drugs.

- *Antioxidants.* During chemo, should you or shouldn't you? This is a controversial topic. Some evidence suggests that they may protect cancer cells, while some evidence suggests otherwise. More research comes out daily—on this issue and on integrative cancer therapies in general. Refer to the Resources section for additional ways to sort through the enormous amount of information about this disease, find out what works and what doesn't, and help you and your doctor to come to the best possible treatment plan for you.

COLCHICINE

This medicine is used to treat gout, a form of arthritis caused by uric acid collecting in the joints and causing inflammation. Sometimes it is given in combination with another drug, probenecid, which slows down the reabsorption of uric acid by the kidneys, allowing it to safely flow out of the body with the urine. Probenecid has no known nutrient depletions.

Action: Colchicine acts as an anti-inflammatory, reducing pain and inflammation that are the main symptoms of gout.

Side effects: The usual drug regimens for gouty arthritis can cause side effects like nausea, vomiting, diarrhea, or abdominal pain, so it's important to strive for overall good nutrition and a high-potency multivitamin if you are being treated for this disease.

Nutrients depleted: Beta-carotene, folic acid, magnesium, potassium, sodium, and vitamin B_{12}.

Needed supplements:

- **Beta-carotene:** Take beta-carotene along with other antioxidants. Beta-carotene is one of a group of nutrients called *carotenoids*, antioxidant plant chemicals that lend color to fruits and vegetables. Alpha-carotene, lutein, zeaxanthin, and lycopene are also carotenoids. Beta-carotene and alpha-carotene can be turned into vitamin A, which is important for the health of the eyes and the nervous system.

   Antioxidants naturally complement one another, and taking one by itself in high doses can actually increase free-radical damage. Your best bet for restoring levels of carotenes is to boost your fruit and vegetable intake—which could help get rid of your gout, too! Put as many naturally bright colors into each meal and snack as you can, and augment with concentrated green food supplements as powders or capsules.

- **Folic acid:** 400 mcg daily.
- **Magnesium:** 250 mg daily.
- **Potassium:** 100 mg daily. Potassium is a mineral abundant in most diets; to make sure you're getting enough, check to see that your multivitamin has around 100 mg per daily dose.
- **Sodium:** As advised by your doctor. This mineral is abundant in most modern diets but if you've been on a sodium-restricted diet, you could run into problems. Speak to your doctor about your adding salt back in as natural a form as possible, such as sea salt.
- **Vitamin B$_{12}$:** 500–1,000 mcg daily. If you suspect that you are low in B$_{12}$, take a sublingual (under the tongue) form. That way it bypasses your digestive system and is absorbed directly into the bloodstream.

Review the dietary recommendations in Chapter 2 for more on adding a greater variety of colorful vegetables into your diet.

CORTICOSTEROIDS

Corticosteroids like prednisone, prednisolone, betamethasone, budenoside, triamcinolone, cortisone, and methylprednisone are miracle drugs. They can be used short-term for acute conditions such as poison ivy or other allergic reactions, and this doesn't pose risk of nutrient depletions. Long-term use is another story.

These medications, when truly needed, can be lifesaving, but taking them over long periods does pose substantial risk. They are used long-term for autoimmune conditions such as rheumatoid arthritis (RA), Crohn's disease, ulcerative colitis, and lupus to reduce inflammation. Corticosteroids may also be needed for severe asthma, to keep the airway open; for allergic rashes such as poison ivy, poison oak, or for a rash that comes from exposure to an irritating chemical; after organ transplant recipients to prevent rejection of the new organ; for adrenal insufficiency, where the adrenal glands are not producing enough hormones; or in cancer patients to reduce pain caused caused by swelling of tumors.

Action: Just like the corticosteroids made in the adrenal glands, they act as anti-inflammatories.

Side effects: Insomnia, indigestion, increased appetite, weight gain, mental problems including psychosis, unwanted immune suppression.

Nutrients depleted: Calcium, folic acid, magnesium, potassium, selenium, vitamins D and E, and zinc.

Needed supplements:

- **Calcium:** 1,000–1,200 mg daily.

- **Magnesium:** 400–600 mg daily.

- **Potassium:** 100 mg daily.

- **Selenium:** 50–200 mcg daily. Selenium is a trace mineral that is depleted in modern diets. Low intake is linked to greater risk of heart disease and cancer. It is an essential ingredient in your body's anti-oxidant system. Selenium has been the subject of intense study for its anti-cancer, immune-boosting, heart-protective effects. Your multi-vitamin should offer adequate selenium to replace this mineral.

- **Vitamin D:** 1,000 IU daily.

- **Vitamin E:** 400 IU daily.

- **Zinc:** 25–50 mg daily.

- **Other nutrients:** See pages 93–94 in Chapter 5 for other supplements helpful for inflammatory conditions.

DIGOXIN

Digoxin, derived from the foxglove plant, is used to treat heartbeat irregularities (arrhythmias), generally atrial fibrillation and atrial flutter—both of which are dangerous conditions. While formerly used to treat congestive heart failure, more modern drugs (diuretics, ACE inhibitors) are usually used for this condition today.

Action: Digoxin (brand names Lanoxin, Lanoxicaps) works by making the heart muscle contract more forcefully. It also decreases conduction of the electrical signal that causes it to beat, which slows down the dangerously fast heart rhythm.

Side effects: Nausea, vomiting, diarrhea, dizziness, headache, weakness, slow heart rate, blurred vision, and mental changes. Low blood potassium or magnesium levels and high calcium levels can increase digoxin toxicity and produce serious heart rhythm disturbances. Digoxin interacts dangerously with other cardiovascular medications, such as quinidine, verapamil, and amiodarone, and beta blockers.

Nutrients depleted: Calcium, magnesium, phosphorus, and vitamin B_1.

Needed supplements:

- **Calcium:** 1,000–1,200 mg daily.
- **Magnesium:** 400–600 mg daily.
- **Phosphorus:** 700 mg daily.
- **Vitamin B_1:** 25 mg daily.
- **Other supplements:** See pages 78–79 in Chapter 4 for other supplements helpful for cardiovascular conditions.

ISONIAZID

This drug is used to treat tuberculosis, or to prevent it in people who are exposed to the disease. Isoniazid is sold under the brand names Laniazid Oral and Nydrazid Injection.

Action: It's used in combination with other drugs to kill the bacteria called *mycobacteria* that cause tuberculosis.

Side effects: Rarely, severe liver problems that lead to hepatitis; more commonly, stomach upset, dizziness, heartburn, or nausea.

Nutrients depleted: Calcium, folic acid, vitamins B_3 and B_6, and vitamin D.

Needed supplements:

- **Calcium:** 1,000–1,200 mg daily.
- **Folic acid:** 400–800 mcg
- **Vitamin B_3:** 25 mg daily.
- **Vitamin B_6:** 10–50 mg daily. Vitamin B_6 is strongly depleted by this drug, and this depletion is believed to be the reason for a common side effect: nerve damage in the hands and feet. Supplementing isoniazid with this vitamin is recommended even by mainstream medicine. See pages 48–52 for more on the B vitamins).
- **Vitamin D:** 1,000 mg daily.

LEVODOPA (L-DOPA)

This medication is used to treat Parkinson's disease (PD). It contains two synthetic forms of the neurotransmitter dopamine (levodopa plus carbidopa), which declines dramatically in Parkinson's sufferers. Without dopamine, muscles become progressively "frozen," and without the drug, he or she may not be able to move at all.

Action: In Parkinson's, there is a loss of dopamine-producing cells in the brain. Levodopa supplies the missing dopamine, allowing movement to be restored to varying degrees.

Side effects: L-Dopa greatly prolongs survival in people with PD, but that comes with liabilities, including the characteristic "thrashing" you might have seen in the now-infamous political ad with Parkinson's patient Michael J. Fox. This side effect is called *dyskinesia*. Other side effects include nausea, vomiting, heart rhythm disturbances, restlessness, and confusion.

Nutrients depleted: Potassium, SAMe, and vitamin B_6.

Needed supplements:

- **Antioxidants:** High levels of antioxidants are also useful in treating PD, which may be due to excessive exposure to toxins such as pesticides in susceptible individuals. Talk with your doctor about this.
- **CoQ_{10}:** 360–1,200 mg daily. No specific research has been done to show that Parkinson's drugs deplete CoQ_{10}. We do know, however, that CoQ_{10} is low in PD patients. A study found that CoQ_{10} supplements slowed down the disease in patients with early-stage PD. The greatest benefit was found at a dose of 1,200 mg per day; less improvement was seen at 300 and 600 mg.
- **Potassium:** L-Dopa may cause an increased urinary loss of potassium in some Parkinson's patients. Use the dose recommended in the multinutrient program on page 32, or more if your doctor recommends it.
- **Vitamin B_6:** 50 mg daily. This vitamin may accelerate the metabolism of levodopa, but this can be overcome by adding carbidopa (Sinemet).

METHOTREXATE

The toxic, powerful drug methotrexate (Folex PFS, Rheumatrex, Trexall) is used for cancer chemotherapy and to treat rheumatoid arthritis and psoriasis.

Action: Methotrexate inhibits the synthesis of DNA, the genetic material that gives cells (including cancer cells and rapidly multiplying skin cells that cause psoriasis) instructions about how to grow and reproduce themselves.

Side effects: Mouth sores, altered white blood cell counts, stomach upset, drowsiness, dizziness, headache, hair loss, and itching.

Nutrients depleted: This drug profoundly depletes folic acid, because it interferes with the process that activates this nutrient in the body.

Needed supplements:

- **Folic acid:** Usually, doctors prescribe a much higher than normal dose of 1,000–5,000 mg (1–5 grams) to overcome the depletion, in the form of *leucovorin* (a fast-acting and more potent form of folic acid). In addition, take 500–1,000 mcg of B_{12}, to prevent B_{12} deficiency—which can be masked by folic acid supplementation.

ORAL CONTRACEPTIVES/ ESTROGEN REPLACEMENT THERAPY

These two medications are used at quite different times in a woman's life: the first, to prevent pregnancy or regulate menstrual cycles during the years of fertility; and the second, to deal with hot flashes and other symptoms that can crop up at menopause. Both contain some version of estrogen, which is a depleting drug, and—unless the woman is menopausal and has had a hysterectomy—will always contain some form of progestin, a synthetic version of progesterone. Other forms of hormonal birth control that come in patches or implants also contain these same drugs, and so are likely to cause the same depletions.

Action: These medications are not truly hormone *replacements*. They are synthetic modifications of the hormone molecules that are close enough copies to fool the receptor sites on the cells. Not only are you getting fake hormones that don't do all of the jobs done by the real hormones, but their presence in your body suppresses production of your own hormones—estrogen, progesterone, and even testosterone.

These hormones are considered "reproductive," but each has other roles. Estrogen stimulates mental and physical energy, in addition to breast development and other female characteristics. Progesterone, which is needed for healthy pregnancy, is also calming to the nervous system. Testosterone is essential for energy and libido.

For menopausal symptoms, I'm a strong proponent of bio-identical hormone replacement therapy over conventional, synthetic versions. Bio-identical hormones exactly match what is made by your ovaries, and have the same benefits with fewer risks. You can read more about the advantages of bio-identical estrogen and progesterone (and, for some women, testosterone) in the book I wrote with Kathleen Barnes, *8 Weeks to Vibrant Health* (McGraw-Hill, 2005). They don't deplete nutrients, either.

Unfortunately, there's still no bio-identical oral contraceptive available.

Side effects: *Oral contraceptives* are highly effective, no doubt, but they raise risk of breast and cervical cancers and of cervical dysplasia, the precancerous condition the doctor looks for when doing a Pap smear. This risk is especially high in young women who use the pill starting in adolescence and continue to do so for many years.

Oral contraceptives also increase risk of heart attack and blood clots. Low sex drive on the pill? It's caused by low testosterone, which, in turn, is caused by the synthetic hormones. (They raise a protein in the blood called *sex hormone binding globulin,* which then binds to testosterone and makes the hormone unavailable). Depression on the pill? It's due to depletion of vitamins such as vitamins C and B_6, needed to make the feel-good brain chemicals called neurotransmitters. (For more information on these neurotransmitters, see page 114.)

Healthier ways to prevent pregnancy: the intrauterine device (IUD), condoms, and the rhythm method—which, if you get instruction from a knowledgeable medical practitioner and follow it to the letter, works almost as well as condoms and pills.

Standard Premarin/progestin hormone therapy is linked with increased risk of breast cancer, stroke, and heart attack. Side effects may also include blood clots, leg pain, vision problems, abnormal vaginal bleeding, dizziness, fluid retention, mood changes, fatigue, acne, decreased libido, and hair loss.

Nutrients depleted: Calcium, folic acid, magnesium, vitamins B_2, B_6, B_{12}, vitamin C, and zinc.

Needed supplements:

- **Calcium:** 1,000–1,200 mg daily.
- **Folic acid:** 400–800 mcg daily.
- **Magnesium:** 400–600 mg daily.

- **Vitamin B₂:** 25 mg daily.
- **Vitamin B₆:** 50 mg daily.
- **Vitamin B₁₂:** 500–1,000 mcg daily.
- **Vitamin C:** 500–1,000 mg
- **Zinc:** 25–50 mg daily.

OSTEOPOROSIS DRUGS

Alendronate (Fosamax) and risedronate (Actonel) belong to the *bisphosphonate* class of drugs. Bisphosphonates are widely prescribed to prevent and treat osteoporosis and to prevent fractures. Some pills are taken daily, and others once a week or once monthly.

Action: These medications slow bone loss by slowing the action of *osteoclasts*, cells that break down bone. As we age, osteoclasts can break bone down faster than *osteoblasts* build new bone from calcium, magnesium, and other minerals.

Side effects: Possible side effects of bisphosphonates include abdominal pain, anxiety, back pain, belching, bladder irritation, bone disorders and pain, bronchitis, bursitis, cataracts, chest pain, colitis, constipation, depression, diarrhea, difficulty breathing, dizziness, dry eyes, eye infection, flu-like symptoms, gas, headache, high blood pressure, infection, insomnia, itching, joint disorders and pain, leg cramps, muscle pain, abdominal pain, muscle weakness, nausea, pneumonia, rash, ringing in ears, sinus problems, sore throat, stomach bleeding, stuffy or runny nose, swelling, tendon problems, tumor, ulcers, urinary tract infection, vertigo, vision problems, and weakness.

A newly discovered, rare, but severe side effect is *osteonecrosis* of the jaw (ONJ), a disfiguring and disabling condition where, after minor trauma such as a tooth extraction, the jaw bones suffer literal bone death, becoming infected and rotten.

Bisphosphonates have to be taken without food, and nothing can be eaten for thirty minutes after swallowing them. Patients are cautioned not to lie down after swallowing the pill and to take it with plenty of water because the medicine is caustic enough to burn the esophagus.

It's widely accepted in medical circles that bisphosphonates do build bone—but that the bone they build is brittle and more prone to fracture than healthy bone built up through the right lifestyle choices.

The *selective estrogen receptor modulators* (SERMs) are another drug class for osteoporosis, which includes tamoxifen and raloxifene (Evista). Although they do improve bone density, they pose a significant risk of blood clots.

Nutrients depleted: Because bisphosphonates push calcium into the bones, blood levels of this mineral—which also plays a role in muscle contraction and relaxation—can be depleted if dietary intake is too low. Essentially, these bone-building drugs have a calcium-depleting effect.

Needed supplements: Take calcium, magnesium, boron, vitamin D and vitamin K to ensure that you have enough of these minerals to fulfill all of their roles in the body. Any woman approaching or in menopause should use these supplements, plus a couple more to really get ahead of the curve and prevent osteoporosis; see below.

Discuss the extent of your bone loss with your doctor, and see whether you can try taking the following steps to promote better bone density, instead of taking a medication:

- **Boron:** 3 mg daily.
- **Calcium:** 1,000–1,200 mg daily.
- **Magnesium:** 400–600 mg daily.
- **Strontium** (shown to help calcium to build better bone): 340 mg twice a day between meals, taken separately from calcium.
- **Vitamin D:** at least 800 IU daily.
- **Vitamin K:** 30–100 mcg daily.
- **Weight-bearing exercise,** including some form of cardiovascular workout plus strength training.
- **Eat some soy every day,** preferably fermented (tempeh, miso). Unfermented soy milk and tofu will not have the same estrogen-like strengthening effect on bone.

Bio-identical hormone replacement (possibly, including estrogen in the form of estradiol and/or estriol; and definitely including natural progesterone) is very effective for maintenance of bone mass in post-menopausal women. Estrogens slow down osteoclasts (bone-destroying cells), while progesterone stimulates osteoblasts (bone-building cells).

Every young woman needs to be aware that her young years are crucial for building optimal bone mass. Studies have shown that a significant percentage of young women are already at risk for developing osteoporosis later in life because they've failed to build up their bones. Exercise, calcium/magnesium/vitamin D, and a good diet are crucial in the teens and early twenties. Drinking soda pop can deplete calcium by introducing too much phosphorus into the body.

SULFASALAZINE

Sulfasalazine (Azulfidine, Azulfidine EN-tabs) is used to treat rheumatoid arthritis and ulcerative colitis.

Action: It acts as an anti-inflammatory in both ulcerative colitis and rheumatoid arthritis by reducing pro-inflammatory, hormone-like messengers called prostaglandins.

Side effects: Side effects include headache, nausea, vomiting, and diarrhea.

Nutrients depleted: Like methotrexate (see above), this drug has a direct folate-depleting effect. It also depletes vitamins B_6 and B_{12}.

Needed supplements:
- **Folic acid:** Supplementing with up to 1 gram (800 mcg) of folic acid daily should help prevent folic acid deficiency.
- **Vitamin B_6:** 50 mg daily.
- **Vitamin B_{12}:** 1,000 mcg daily.

Certainly, we're all grateful for medicines when we really need them, despite the reality of risks and side effects. A powerful plan to replenish nutrients known to be depleted by those drugs, combined with the use of other nutrients scientifically shown to be helpful for your condition, can give you even greater control of your path back to health.

NINE

A Delicate Balance: Concluding Thoughts

So far, we've looked in-depth at the drugs that are most likely to be in your medicine cabinet. You've learned about natural solutions to the underlying causes of your health problems. In many cases, this will allow you—with the help of your doctor—to reduce the number or dosages of prescriptions you are taking, or eliminate them altogether. Replenishing the nutrients depleted by the drugs you take could make a big difference in your quality of life and long-term health.

This is especially true if you take two, three, or even four or more drugs on an ongoing basis. In this chapter, you'll find special pointers to help you reduce your risks and enhance the benefits of your medications.

In this final wrap-up chapter, I will also share a few more words of advice about making your integrative health-care program as safe and effective as possible. You'll learn about using your doctor and pharmacist as resources, and about finding a doctor who supports and improves upon your integrative health-care path.

POLYPHARMACY: WHAT YOU SHOULD KNOW

Polypharmacy—the use of three or more drugs simultaneously—is quite common, particularly in people over sixty-five and those with serious or chronic conditions. Even if you take only one prescription medication, you'll probably feel the need to add in one or two over-the-counter (OTC) medicines from time to time. Even medicinal herbs can interact harmfully with prescriptions or OTC drugs. More and more drugs, together with herbal preparations, are available over the counter, with no consultation or prescription required.

Let's say you're taking a couple of prescription drugs . . . you add a few herbs and a dose or two of Tylenol here and there . . . and, of course, your nightly beer or glass of red wine (or two). You're playing a dangerous game with your health—a game that has killed some well-known people. Remember Anna Nicole Smith? Hers is far from the only example where young, generally healthy people—who didn't think that the combination of chemicals they were consuming would hurt them—ended up in the hospital or dead.

Your body is an amazing machine, and it can bounce back from a lot of abuse. Appreciate its delicate balance and don't push it to extremes by piling on medicines and herbs (which can act like drugs) without a physician consultation. Here are some other pointers to help you get the most out of your prescriptions, if you use two or more on a regular basis:

- Know your meds well: what they're for, the generic and brand names, how they affect your body, and what side effects, including nutrient depletions, you might expect. Each drug has its own description on the company's website. It includes side effects and at least some nutrient depletions. Refer to these sites and familiarize yourself completely with any drugs you take regularly.

- Keep a clear written list of all of your medications, including dosage, schedules, and the day on which you first took them. Track your intake daily, in a notebook or on a calendar. It's easy to forget what you've taken, and it gets worse as you age. Caregivers: this is where you step in and keep records.

- If you want to consume alcohol, make sure that it's compatible with your medications.

- Allow your doctor to monitor you closely any time he or she adds a new medication.

- Talk to your doctor or to a pharmacist before adding any OTC drug or herbal supplement to your regimen, and keep each of your doctors informed about what drugs and nutrients you are taking.

- Have all your doctors talk to each other. Symptoms from different underlying conditions can be the same, and two doctors may end up treating them differently, overloading you with prescriptions. One recent example in my own practice: Iris was depressed and fatigued; one doctor tried to treat her depression with an antidepressant (but couldn't use Prozac because it fueled her anxiety); he prescribed Lexapro at 15 milligrams (mg) a day, which made her too tired, so cut the dose back to 10 mg. She was still tired, but he blamed it on her thyroid and told her to see her endocrinologist. The latter, however, told her it was likely still a side effect of the Lexapro. She felt caught in the middle of these specialists. Was it her thyroid? Her neurotransmitters? Some other hormones? Remember that doctors may not talk to one another to find the root cause of your health problems—unless you encourage them to do so. Fortunately, I stepped in, tested her across the board, and found a solution that worked. I conferred with her other doctors to create a comprehensive get-well plan for her.

• Buy all your prescriptions from one pharmacy and get to know the pharmacist. Your pharmacist is an excellent resource, and can give you descriptive handouts along with each prescription. Pharmacists can also be consulted with specific questions. They keep an eye on your prescription list to avoid excessive prescribing, which can happen when several doctors are unaware of each other's prescriptions. Your pharmacist is always on the lookout for dangerous drug interactions.

• Even if you need multiple medications, keep in mind that you will benefit a great deal from the basics recommended in Chapter 2. That's the foundation that can build your health back to where you might not need so many medications after all!

FINDING AN INTEGRATIVE MEDICINE DOCTOR

Many times throughout this book, I've recommended that you consult with your doctor when starting a new nutritional supplement. Unfortunately, some physicians will be less than supportive when you bring up this topic. This may be due to ignorance—after all, your doctor has to keep up with the research on drugs, procedures, and diagnoses, and isn't likely to have the time or energy to bone up on nutrition. Or it may be because of misguided notions about the scientific support for nutritional supplementation in people who are depleted by prescription drugs.

If you are truly committed to embracing both medications and vitamin/diet/lifestyle approaches—and you should, as this increases your chances of success by capitalizing on the strengths of both—and your doctor isn't interested in helping you out, you might consider seeking out a more supportive medical practitioner. More and more of my colleagues are taking an active interest in this area, and I find that many of the finest conventional medical doctors are beginning to read the literature and incorporate this new information.

Integrative medicine combines conventional and complementary therapies that are based in science. *Functional medicine* is another term used to describe this field, which incorporates the use of nutrition and nutritional supplements. Based on the particular needs of the individual, it requires that the doctor and patient be partners in care. Research shows that nearly one in three Americans is seeking out integrative care, and many medical schools have begun to include it in their curriculum.

You may decide to look for an integrative M.D. or D.O. (Doctor of Osteopathy, who takes all of the coursework an M.D. does, with additional training about the interrelationship between the body's structure and function). In the Resources section, you'll find listings of different organizations that maintain databases of doctors who support the integration of natural therapies with mainstream medicine. These organizations have Web pages and phone numbers that will make your search easier.

Take your time seeking out a doctor that you relate to and can trust. Ask friends and family to make recommendations. Your relationship with your physician is of primary importance in your life, so it's worth making a well-researched choice.

Your doctor should be able to help you reevaluate your need for your current medications, and perhaps reduce the number and dose as you integrate smart nutrient supplementation and adjustments into your diet and lifestyle.

FINAL THOUGHTS FOR EDUCATED PATIENTS

New discoveries are likely to be made about nutrients depleted by prescription drugs, as well as side effects, drug interactions, drug/nutrient interactions, and risks. You can use the Web to stay up to date on these issues. Refer to the Resources for this chapter (Chapter 9) for sites useful in this regard. If you don't use the Web, it's even more important for you to stay in touch with your pharmacist and medical team to keep current.

You may take a medication or have a condition that wasn't covered in this book. If so, keep in mind that I tried to include every commonly used medicine that depletes nutrients, but that you may need more information if a drug you use or a condition that affects you isn't in these pages. The Resources section for this chapter will give you options for getting the information you need.

As you embark upon your new integrative health program, remember that natural treatments require more time and patience to bring results. Prescription drugs can work so quickly, and we've become conditioned to expect rapid results from supplements and herbs, too. I encourage you to allow at least a month or two for any natural treatment to kick in and improve your health. It takes longer because these treatments go deeper, addressing underlying health imbalances, rather than simply reducing your symptoms. If you want to heal, not just feel better today (at the price of depending on a prescription drug long term), you'll find it's worth the wait.

In the end, be respectful of the power of prescription medications, both to heal and to harm. By educating yourself about possible nutrient depletions, side effects, and drug interactions, you will be in the best position possible to take advantage of the positive effects of your medications. And by supplementing accordingly, beyond just the level of the depletions, you are giving yourself a chance for true healing and optimal health. You deserve it.

Resources

For updates and additional resources, check out www.drcass.com. You can also email me at www.drcass.com. Please note: Contact information is subject to change.

Chapter 1: What You Should Know about Drugs

Books

Abramson, John, M.D. *Overdosed America*. New York, NY: Harper Perennial, 2005.

Angell, Marcia, M.D. *The Truth About the Drug Companies: How They Deceive Us and What to Do About It*. New York, NY: Random House, 2004.

Cohen, Jay, M.D. *Over Dose: The Case Against the Drug Companies*. New York, NY: Tarcher/Putnam, 2001.

Websites

Applied Nutrition's Drug-Nutrient Workshop—www.nutritionworkshop.com: This website allows you to search for potential reactions between drugs, herbs, vitamins, minerals, and other nutritional supplements.

Center for Food-Drug Interaction Research and Education—www.druginteractioncenter.org: New online tool with patient section to check interactions established by the University of Florida and Tufts University School of Medicine.

Consumer Reports Best Buy Drugs—www.crbestbuydrugs.org: A useful site for checking out a drug's side effects, and often, information on nutrient depletions.

Institute for Safe Medication Practices—www.ismp.org: Provides timely medication safety information and allows you to report adverse drug reactions in confidence to the FDA and manufacturer.

MedicineNet's *MedTerms Medical Dictionary*—www.medterms.com/script/main/hp.asp.

Chapter 2: You Hold the Keys to Your Health

Books

Appleton, Nancy, Ph.D. *Lick the Sugar Habit*. Garden City Park, NY: Avery, 2001.

Berthold-Bond, Annie. *Home Enlightenment: Practical, Earth-Friendly Advice for Creating a Nurturing, Healthy, and Toxin-Free Home and Lifestyle*. New York, NY: Rodale Books, 2007.

Cordain, Loren, Ph.D., *The Paleo Diet: Lose Weight and Get Healthy by Eating the Food You Were Designed to Eat*. New York, NY: Wiley, 2002.

Gittleman, Ann Louise, Ph.D. *Fat Flush Cookbook*. New York: NY: McGraw-Hill, 2003.

Gittleman, Ann Louise, Ph.D. *Fat Flush Plan*. New York: NY: McGraw-Hill, 2002.

Heber, David, M.D., Ph.D. *What Color is Your Diet*. New York, NY: HarperCollins, 2001.

Herb Research Foundation. *Best Herbs for Healing*. New York, NY: Prentice Hall, 2007.

Hyman, Mark, M.D. and Mark Lippnis, M.D. *Ultraprevention: The 6-Week Plan That Will Make Your Healthy for Life.*New York, NY: Atria, 2005.

Natow, Annette, and Jo-Ann Heslin. *The Protein Counter*. New York, NY: Pocket Books, 2003.

Rowe, Barbara, M.P.H., R.D., L.D., C.N.S.D. *Anti-Inflammatory Foods for Health: Hundreds of Ways to Incorporate Omega-3 Rich, Fat-Fighting Foods into Your Diet*. Beverly, MA: Fair Winds Press, 2008.

Sears, Barry, Ph.D. *What to Eat in the Zone*. New York, NY: HarperCollins, 2003.

Sears, Barry, Ph.D. with Bill Lawren. *Enter the Zone*. New York, NY: Regan Books, 1995.

Woodruff, Sandra, M.S., R.D., L.D.N. *Secrets of Good-Carb Low Carb Living*. New York, NY: Avery, 2004.

Zimmerman, Marcia, M.Ed., C.N. *Eat Your Colors*. New York, NY: Owl Books, 2001.

DVDs

You: On a Diet Workout—This DVD comes from Drs. Mehmet Oz and Michael Roizen, authors of the terrific books *You: The Owner's Manual* (New York, NY: Collins, 2005) and *You: On a Diet* (New York, NY: Free Press, 2006); it's a straightforward, no-frills, comprehensive workout that you can do at home in your socks in twenty minutes.

Newsletters

Naturally Well Today: Monthly newsletter about natural health by naturopathic physician, Marcus Laux; for more information, see www.DrMarcusLaux.com.

*Nutrition News:*Reliable, well-researched monthly nutrition newsletter on health and nutrition in a user-friendly format written and published by Siri Khalsa since 1976; for more information, see www.nutritionnews.com.

Websites

American Botanical Council—www.herbalgram.org: Independent, nonprofit research and education organization; great resource for the latest accurate information about herbal medicines.

Consumer Lab—www.consumerlab.com: Independent testing and evaluation of nutritional supplements; a useful tool for choosing the best quality for your money. Requires a subscription, but well worth the nominal fee.

Council for Responsible Nutrition (CRN)—www.crnusa.org: Trade association representing dietary-supplement-industry ingredient suppliers and manufacturers; supports high-quality standards under good manufacturing practices (GMP).

Linus Pauling Institute Micronutrient Information Center—http://lpi.oregonstate.edu/ infocenter: An up-to-date database of research-based information on various nutrients.

My Vitamins Matter—www.myvitaminsmatter.com: A website hosted by USP-certified supplement manufacturers; it is designed to help consumers to sort out the truth from the fictions in the supplement marketplace, and to offer easy-to-understand, current information about nutritional supplements.

National Institutes of Health (NIH) Vitamin and Mineral Supplement Fact Sheets—http://ods.od.nih.gov/Health_Information/Vitamin_and_Mineral_Supplement_Fact_She ets.aspx: NIH fact sheets on vitamins and minerals.

Seafood Choices Alliance—www.seafoodchoices.org: Check this site to ensure that you are choosing seafood that is sustainable and as nontoxic as possible.

Website of medical writer and diabetes consultant David Mendosa—www.mendosa. com: Includes an extensive listing of glycemic indices of foods and information about diabetes.

Chapter 3: Prescriptions for Blood Sugar Balance

Books

Braly, James, M.D. and Patrick Holford. *The H Factor: Homocysteine, the Best Single Indicator of Whether You Are Likely to Live Longer or Die Young.*Laguna Beach, CA: Basic Health Publications, 2003.

Brand-Miller, Jennie, Ph.D., Kaye Foster-Powell, Stephen Colagiuri, and Alan Barclay. *The New Glucose Revolution for Diabetes: The Definitive Guide to Managing Diabetes and Prediabetes Using the Glycemic Index.* New York, NY: Marlowe & Company, 2007.

DVDs

Raw for 30 Days by Mark Perlmutter. A moving documentary film about six advanced diabetics on a vegan, organic, raw food diet for a month, supervised by medical staff at the Tree of Life Rejuvenation Center in Patagonia, AZ, with excellent results. Release date: Spring 2008. A compendium DVD is also being produced about the program to reverse diabetes; for more information, see www.Rawfor30Days.com.

Websites

Diabetes Information/Diabetes Pills—www.fda.gov/diabetes/pills.html: Website from the Food and Drug Administration on diabetes medications.

Homocysteine.net—www.homocysteine.net: A wealth of information.

Chapter 4: Prescriptions for Cardiovascular Health

Books

Challem, Jack. *The Inflammation Syndrome: The Complete Nutritional Program to Prevent and Reverse Heart Disease, Diabetes, Arthritis, Allergies, and Asthma.* (New York, NY: Wiley, 2003.

Cohen, Jay, M.D. *What You Must Know About Statin Drugs and Their Natural Alternatives.*New York, NY: Square One, 2004.

Graveline, Duane, M.D. *Statin Drugs: Side Effects and The Misguided War on Cholesterol.* Duane Graveline, 2006.

Websites

International Coenzyme Q_{10} Association—www.coenzymeq10.it/home.html: Provides articles, research summaries, and study citations on CoQ_{10}.

Chapter 5: Prescriptions for Arthritis

Books

Cass, Hyla, M.D. *User's Guide to Vitamin C.* Laguna Beach, CA: Basic Health Publications, 2003.

Sarno, John, M.D. *Healing Back Pain: TheMindbody Connection.* New York, NY: Grand Central Publishing, 1991.

Sarno, John, M.D. *The Mindbody Prescription: Healing the Body, Healing the Pain.* New York, NY: Grand Central Publishing, 1999.

Teitelbaum, Jacob, M.D. *Painfree 1-2-3.* New York, NY: McGraw-Hill, 2005.

Websites

About.com—www.arthritis.about.com: Excellent resource on arthritis.

WebMD's Arthritis Health Center—http://arthritis.webmd.com: An excellent resource for general information on arthritis and medications used to treat it.

Chapter 6: Prescriptions for Digestive Function

Books

Crook, William, M.D. *The Yeast Connection: A Medical Breakthrough.* Newton, MA: Professional Books/Future Health, 1989.

Martin, Jeanne Marie, with Zoltan Roma, M.D. *Complete Candida Yeast Guidebook: Everything You Need to Know About Prevention, Treatment & Diet.* New York, NY: Three Rivers Press, 2003.

Rogers, Sherry. *No More Heartburn: Stop the Pain in 30 Days—Naturally.* New York NY: Kensington, 2000.

Websites

The World's Healthiest Foods—www.whfoods.org/genpage.php?tname=diet&dbid=7: This part of the website of the George Matelijan Foundation contains a simple, easy-to-follow description of a food allergy elimination diet.

Chapter 7: Prescriptions for Psychological Health

Books

Breggin, Peter, M.D., and David Cohen, Ph.D. *Your Drug May Be Your Problem: How and Why to Stop Taking Psychiatric Medications.* Reading, MA: Perseus Books, 2007; see also, www.breggin.com.

Brown, Richard and Carol Colman. *Stop Depression Now: SAM-e, The Breakthrough*

Supplement that Works as Well as Prescription Drugs. New York, NY: Berkley Trade, 2000.

Cass, Hyla, M.D., and Kathleen Barnes. *8 Weeks to Vibrant Health.* New York, NY: McGraw-Hill, 2004.

Cass, Hyla, M.D., and Patrick Holford. *Natural Highs: Feel Good All the Time.* New York, NY, Penguin Group, 2002.

Glenmullen, Joseph, M.D. *The Antidepressant Solution: A Step-by-Step Guide to Safely Overcoming Antidepressant Withdrawal, Dependence, and Addiction.* New York, NY: Free Press, 2006.

Glenmullen, Joseph, M.D. *Prozac Backlash: Overcoming the Dangers of Prozac, Zoloft, Paxil, and Other Antidepressants with Safe, Effective Alternatives.* New York, NY: Simon & Schuster, 2000.

Holford, Patrick. *Optimum Nutrition for Your Mind.* Laguna Beach, CA: Basic Health Publications, 2004.

Stoll, Andrew, Stoll, M.D. *The Omega-3 Connection: The Groundbreaking Antidepression Diet and Brain Program.* New York, NY: Free Press, 2002.

Websites

About.com—www.depression.about.com: Lots of great information on all aspects of depression and its treatment.

Cognitive Behavior Therapy (CBT) website—www.cognitivetherapy.com: Provides resources, articles, and a database of CBT professionals.

Consumer Reports Best Buy Drugs—www.crbestbuydrugs.org/PDFs/Antidepressants _update.pdf: Good report comparing effectiveness and safety of antidepressants.

International Guide to the World of Alternative Mental Health—http://alternativemen talhealth.com: Resource for non-drug approaches for mental health.

National Alliance on Mental Illness (NAMI)—http://nami.org: Nation's largest grass-roots mental health organization dedicated to improving the lives of persons living with serious mental illness and their families.

National Institute of Mental Health—www.nimh.nih.gov: Excellent resource on all aspect of mental health and illness.

Chapter 8: Prescriptions for Other Conditions

Books

Alschuler, Lise, N.D., and Karolyn Gazelle. *Alternative Medicine Magazine's Definitive Guide to Cancer: An Integrated Approach for Treatment and Healing.* Berkeley, CA: Celestial Arts, 2007.

Hyla Cass, M.D., and Kathleen Barnes. *8 Weeks to Vibrant Health: A Woman's Take-Charge Program to Correct Imbalances, Reclaim Energy, and Restore Well-Being.* New York, NY: McGraw-Hill, 2005.

Labriola, Dan. *Complementary Cancer Therapies: Combining Traditional and Alternative Approaches for the Best Possible Outcome.* Roseville, CA: Prima Lifestyles, 2000.

Rountree, Robert, M.D., and Carol Colman. *Immunotics: A Revolutionary Way to Fight Infection, Beat Chronic Illness, and Stay Well.* New York, NY: G.P. Putnam's Sons, 2000.

Newsletters

*Women's Health Letter:*Nutritionist and author Nan Fuchs's monthly newsletter for anything you'd like to know about natural approaches women's health; for more information, see www.womenshealthletter.com.

Websites

Cancer Treatment Centers of America—www.cancercenter.com: Network of cancer treatment hospitals that encourage use of complementary and alternative medicine (CAM) approaches, along with conventional cancer therapies.

Cancerdecisions.com—www.cancerdecisions.com: Dr. Ralph W. Moss's website that critically evaluates and contrasts both conventional and alternative cancer therapies. Offers cancer treatment tips, free newsletter, and educational resources for health professionals. For an additional fee, patients can purchase *The Moss Reports* (www.ralph-moss.com), an individualized summary of various options applicable to their cancer, culled from a database of numerous cancer conditions.

International Academy of Compounding Pharmacists—www.iacprx.org: Resource for a comprehensive list of compounding pharmacies.

National Cancer Institute, Complementary and Alternative Medicine Treatment Options —www.cancernet.nci.nih.gov/cancertopics/treatment/cam.

Oncology Channel—www.oncologychannel.com: Information on conventional cancer treatments.

Chapter 9: A Delicate Balance

Books

Ettinger, Alan, M.D., and Deborah Weisbrot, M.D. *The Essential Patient Handbook: Getting the Health Care You Need From Doctors Who Know.* New York, NY: Demos Medical Publishing, 2004.

Hoffman, Ronald, M.D. *How to Talk to Your Doctor.* Laguna Beach, CA: Basic Health Publications, 2006.

Websites

American Association of Naturopathic Physicians—www.naturopathic.org: Free online search for naturopathic physicians in your area.

American Board of Holistic Medicine—www.holisticboard.org: Free referrals to more than 650 M.D.s and D.O.s who are board-certified holistic physicians.

Institute for Functional Medicine—www.functionalmedicine.org: Free online search for functional medicine doctors in your area.

National Center for Complementary and Alternative Medicine (NCCAM)—http://nccam.nih.gov: Federal government's lead agency for scientific research on complementary and alternative medicine.

References

Introduction

Centers for Disease Control and Statistics. "Health, United States, 2006." www.cdc.gov/nchs/data/hus/hus06.pdf#093.

Chapter 1

Lazarou J, BH Pomeranz, PN Corey. "Incidence of adverse drug reactions in hospitalized patients: a meta-analysis of prospective studies." *Journal of the American Medical Association* Apr 15, 1998; 279(15): 1200–1205.

Moore T, MR Cohen, and C Furber. "Serious adverse drug events reported to the Food and Drug Administration, 1998–2005." *Archives of Internal Medicine* 2007; 167(16): 1752–1759.

Chapter 2

Casagrande SS, Y Wang, C Anderson, et al. "Have Americans increased their fruit and vegetable intake? trends between 1988 and 2002." *American Journal of Preventive Medicine* 2007; 32(4): 257–263.

Chapter 3

Barringer TA, JK Kirk, et al. "Effect of a multivitamin and mineral supplement on infection and quality of life: a randomized, double-blind, placebo-controlled trial." *Annals of Internal Medicine* Mar 4, 2003; 138: 365-371.

Cole BF, et al. "Folic acid for the prevention of colorectal adenomas: a randomized clinical trial." *Journal of the American Medical Association* June 6, 2007; 297(21): 2351–2359.

Dormandy JA, B Charbonnel, DJ Eckland, et al. "Secondary prevention of macrovascular events in patients with type 2 diabetes in the PROactive study (PROspective pioglitAzone Clinical Trial In macroVascular Events): a randomised controlled trial." *Lancet* 2005; 366: 1279–1289.

Hammes HP, D Xueliang, D Edelstein, et al. "Benfotiamine blocks three major pathways of hyperglycemic damage and prevents experimental diabetic retinopathy." *Nature Medicine* Mar 2003; 9(3): 294–299.

Kobla HV and SL Volpe. "Chromium, exercise, and body composition." *Critical Reviews in Food Science and Nutrition* 2000; 40(4): 291–308.

Nissen SE and K Wolski. "Effect of rosiglitazone on the risk of myocardial infarction and death from cardiovascular causes." *New England Journal of Medicine* May 21, 2007; www.nejm.org.

Thornalley P, et al. "Prevention of incipient diabetic nephropathy by high-dose thiamine and benfotiamine." *Diabetes* 2003; 52(8): 110-120.

Thornalley P, R Babaei-Jadidi, H Ali, et al. "High prevalence of low plasma thiamine concentration in diabetes linked to a marker of vascular disease." *Diabetologia* Aug 2007; 50(8).

"Top 10 generic drugs by units in 2006" *Drug Topics* March 5, 2007.www.drugtopics.com.

Ulrich CM and JD Potter. "Folate and cancer—timing is everything," *Journal of the American Medical Association* June 6, 2007; 297(21): 2408–2409.

Wald D, et al, "Homocysteine and cardiovascular disease: evidence of causality from a meta-analysis," *British Medical Journal* Nov 23, 2002; 325: 1202.

Wellen KE and GS Hotamisligil. "Inflammation, stress, and diabetes." *Journal of Clinical Investigation* 2005; 115(5): 1111–1119.

Zhao-Wei Ting R, C Chun Szeto, M Ho-Ming Chan, et al. "Risk factors of vitamin B_{12} deficiency in patients receiving metformin." *Archives of Internal Medicine* Oct 9, 2006: 1975–1979.

Chapter 4

Aberg F, et al. "Gemfibrozil-induced decrease in serum ubiquinone and alpha- and gamma-tocopherol levels in men with combined hyperlipidaemia." *European Journal of Clinical Investigation* Mar 1998; 28(3): 235–242.

Alfin-Slater, RB and L Aftergood. "Lipids." *Modern Nutrition in Health and Disease*, 6th ed, RS Goodhart and ME Shils, eds. Philadelphia: Lea and Febiger,1980.

ALLHAT Collaborative Research Group. "Major outcomes in high-risk hypertensive patients randomized to angiotensin-converting enzyme inhibitor or calcium channel blocker vs diuretic." *Journal of the American Medical Association* 2002; 288: 2981–2997.

Altschul R, A Hoffer, JD Stephen. "Influence of nicotinic acid on serum cholesterol in man." *Archives of Biochemistry and Biophysics* 1955; 54: 558–559.

Baker, DE Baker and RK Campbell. "Vitamin and mineral supplementation in patients with diabetes mellitus." *The Diabetes Educator* Sept/Oct 1992; 18(5): 420–427.

Bucher, HC, P Hengstler, C Schindler, et al. "N-3 polyunsaturated fatty acids in coronary heart disease: a meta-analysis of randomized controlled trials." *American Journal of Medicine* 2002; 112(4): 298–304.

Harris TB. "Associations of elevated interleukin-6 and C-reactive protein levels with mortality in the elderly." *American Journal of Medicine* May 1999; 106(5): 506–512.

Davidson, MH. "Mechanisms for the hypotriglyceridemic effect of marine omega-3 fatty acids." *American Journal of Cardiology* Aug 21, 2006; 98(4 Suppl 1): 27–33. Epub: May 26, 2006.

Goldberg AC, RE Ostlund, JH Bateman, et al. "Effect of plant stanol tablets on low-density lipoprotein cholesterol lowering in patients on statin drugs." *American Journal of Cardiology* Feb 2006; 97(3): 376–379.

Guyton, JR, MA Blazing, J Hagar, et al. "Extended-release niacin vs. gemfibrozil for the treatment of low levels of high-density lipoprotein cholesterol." *Archives of Internal Medicine* 2000; 160: 1177–1184.

Leaf, A. *Fundamental & Clinical Pharmacology* Aug 2007;

Mayeda A, et al. "Effects of indirect light and propranolol on melatonin levels in normal human subjects." *Psychiatry Research* Oct 1998; 81(1): 9–17.

Qureshi AA, et al. "Dose-dependent suppression of serum cholesterol by tocotrienol-rich fraction (TRF25) of rice bran in hypercholesterolemic subjects." *Atherosclerosis* Mar 2002; 161(1): 199–207.

Sanders, TA, FR Oakley, GJ Miller, et al. "Influence of n-6 versus n-3 polyunsaturated fatty acids in diets low in saturated fatty acids on plasma lipoproteins and hemostatic factors." *Arteriosclerosis, Thrombosis, and Vascular Biology* 1997; 17(12): 3449–3460.

Savoia C and EL Schiffrin. "Inflammation in hypertension." *Current Opinion in Nephrology and Hypertension* Mar 2006; 15(2): 152–158.

Smith, MM, and F Lifshitz. "Excess fruit juice consumption as a contributing factor in nonorganic failure to thrive." *Pediatrics* Mar 1994; 93(3): 438–443.

Steinlechner S, TS King, TH Champney, et al. "Comparison of the effects of beta-adrenergic agents on pineal serotonin n-acetyltransferase activity and melatonin content in two species of hamsters." *Journal of Pineal Research* 1984; 1(1): 23–30.

Stoschitzky K, et al. "Influence of beta-blockers on melatonin release: gemfibrozil-induced decrease in serum ubiquinone and alpha- and gamma-tocopherol levels in men with combined hyperlipidaemia." *European Journal of Clinical Pharmacology* Apr 1999; 55(2): 111–115.

Studer, M. "Comparative analysis of fish oil and statins." *Archives of Internal Medicine* 2005; 165: 725–730.

Tishler M and S Armon. "Nifedipine-induced hypokalemia." *Drug Intelligence & Clinical Pharmacy* 1986; 20(5): 370–371.

University of California at San Diego Statin Effects Study. "Statin adverse effects." http://medicine.ucsd.edu/ses/adverse_effects.htm (accessed 5/5/07).

Weston Price Foundation. "The skinny on fats." www.karlloren.com/diet/p67.htm.

Zampelas, A, et al. "Fish consumption among healthy adults is associated with decreased levels of inflammatory markers related to cardiovascular disease: the ATTICA study." *Journal of the American College of Cardiology* July 5, 2005; 46(1): 120–124.

Chapter 5

Altman, RD and KC Marcussen. "Effects of a ginger extract on knee pain in patients with osteoarthritis." *Arthritis & Rheumatism* 2001; 44(11): 2531–2538.

Baggott JE, SL Morgan, T Ha, et al. "Inhibition of folate-dependent enzymes by non-steroidal anti-inflammatory drugs," *Biochemical Journal* Feb 15 1992; 282(Pt 1): 197–202.

Baker K, YQ Zhang, J Goggins, et al. "Hypovitaminosis D and its association with muscle strength, pain and physical function in knee osteoarthritis (OA): a 30-month longitudinal, observational study." American College of Rheumatology Meeting, San Antonio, TX, Oct 16–21, 2004; abstract 1755.

Basu TK. "Vitamin C-aspirin interactions." *International Journal for Vitamin and Nutrition Research (Suppl)* 1982; 23: 83–90.

Bliddal, H, A Rosetzsky, P Schlichting, et al. "A randomized, placebo-controlled, crossover study of ginger extracts and ibuprofen in osteoarthritis." *Osteoarthritis Cartilage* 2000; 8(1): 9–12.

Chrubasik S, et al. "Comparison of outcome measures during treatment with the proprietary *Harpagophytum* extract doloteffin in patients with pain in the lower back, knee or hip." *Phytomedicine* 2002; 9: 181–194.

Das N and S Nebioglu. "Vitamin C aspirin interactions in laboratory animals." *Journal of Clinical Pharmacy and Therapeutics* 1992; 17: 343–346.

Lawrence VA, JE Lowenstein, ER Eichner. "Aspirin and folate binding: in vivo and in vitro studies of serum binding and urinary excretion of endogenous folate." *Journal of Laboratory and Clinical Medicine* Jun 1984; 103(6): 944–948.

Loh, HS, K Watters, and CW Wilson. "The effects of aspirin on the metabolic availability of ascorbic acid in human beings." *Journal of Clinical Pharmacology and New Drugs* 1973; 13: 480–486.

"Management of osteoarthritis knee pain: the state of the science." www.medscape.com/viewarticle/536924_4 (accessed 6/18/07).

McAlindon T, et al. "Do antioxidant micronutrients protect against the development and progression of knee osteoarthritis?" *Arthritis & Rheumatism* 1996; 39(4): 648–656.

McAlindon, T and D Felson. "Nutrition: risk factors for osteoarthritis." *Annals of Rheumatic Diseases* 1997; 56: 397–402.

Molloy TP and CW Wilson. "Protein-binding of ascorbic acid 2: interaction with acetylsalicylic acid." *International Journal for Vitamin and Nutrition Research* 1980; 50: 387–392.

Sarno, John. *The Divided Mind: The Epidemic of Mindbody Disorders.* New York, NY: HarperCollins, 2007.

Shaud MA and RJ Cohen. "Effect of aspirin ingestion on ascorbic acid levels in rheumatoid arthritis." *Lancet* 1971; 1: 937–938.

Weatherby, Craig, and Leonid Gordin. *The Arthritis Bible.* Rochester, VT: Healing Arts Press, 1999.

Wigler, I, I Grotto, D Caspi, et al. "The effects of zintona EC (a ginger extract) on symptomatic gonarthritis." *Osteoarthritis Cartilage* 2003; 11(11): 783–789.

Chapter 6

Kennedy, Ron. "Hypochlorhydria." The Doctors' Medical Library. www.med–library.net/content/view/177.

Yang, YX, JD Lewis, S Epstein, et al. "Long-term proton pump inhibitor therapy and risk of hip fracture." *Journal of the American Medical Association* Dec 27, 2006; 296 (24): 2947–2953. PMID 17190895 (retrieved on 1/15/07).

Chapter 7

Abou-Saleh MT and A Coppen. "The biology of folate in depression: implications for nutritional hypotheses of the psychoses." *Journal of Psychiatry Research* 1986; 20(2): 91–101.

Alpert JE and M Fava. "Nutrition and depression: the role of folate." *Nutrition Review* 1997; 5(5): 145–149.

Alpert JE, D Mischoulon, AA Nierenberg, et al. "Nutrition and depression: focus on folate." *Nutrition* 2000; 16(7): 544–546.

Andreassen OA, C Weber, HA Jorgenssen, et al. "Coenzyme Q_{10} does not prevent oral dyskinesias induced by long-term haloperidol therapy of rats," *Pharmacology, Biochemistry, and Behavior* Nov 1999; 64(3): 637–642.

Bernstein AL. "Vitamin B_6 in clinical neurology." *Annals of the New York Academy of Sciences* 1990; 585: 250–260.

Bottiglieri T. "Folate, vitamin B_{12}, and neuropsychiatric disorders." *Nutrition Review* Dec 1996; 54(12): 382–390.

Bottiglieri T, M Laundy, R Crellin, et al. "Homocysteine, folate, methylation, and monoamine metabolism in depression." *Journal of Neurology, Neurosurgery & Psychiatry* Mar 2001; 70(3): 419.

Bressa GM. "S-adenosyl-l-methionine (SAMe) as antidepressant: meta-analysis of clinical studies." *Acta Neurol Scand Suppl* 1994; 154: 7–14.

Diem, SJ and K Saag. *Archives of Internal Medicine.* Jun 25, 2007; 167: 1240–1245.

Elias M. "Study: antidepressant barely better than placebo." *USA Today,* July 7, 2002.

Fava M, JS Borus, JE Alpert, AA Nierenberg, et al. "Folate, vitamin B_{12}, and homocysteine in major depressive disorder." *American Journal of Psychiatry* Mar 1997; 154(3): 426–428.

Gloth FM, W Alam, and B Hollis. "Vitamin D vs broad spectrum phototherapy in the treatment of seasonal affective disorder." *Journal of Nutrition, Health & Aging* 1999; 3(1): 5–7.

Hawkins DR. "Successful prevention of tardive dyskinesia." *Journal of Orthomolecular Medicine* 1989; 4(1): 35–36.

Hintikka J, et al. "High vitamin B_{12} level and good treatment outcome may be associated in major depressive disorder." *Boston Medical Center Psychiatry* Dec 2, 2003; 3: 17.

Hvas AM, et al. "Vitamin B_6 level is associated with symptoms of depression." *Psychotherapy and Psychosomatics* Nov–Dec 2004; 73(6): 340–343.

Kunin RA. "Manganese in dyskinesias."*American Journal of Psychiatry* 1976; 133: 10.

Lansdowne AT and SC Provost. "Vitamin D3 enhances mood in healthy subjects during winter." *Psychopharmacology* (Berl), Feb 1998; 135(4): 319–323.

Madhukar H, M Trivedi, M Fava, et al. "Medication augmentation after the failure of SSRIs for depression." *New England Journal of Medicine* 2006; 354: 1243–1252.

Morris MS, M Fava, PF Jacques, et al. "Depression and folate status in the U.S. population." *Psychotherapy and Psychosomatics* Mar–Apr 2003; 72(2): 59–60.

Norris JP and RE Sams. "More on the use of manganese in dyskinesia." *American Journal of Psychiatry* 1997; 134: 1448.

javascript:PopUpMenu2_Set(Menu9155210);Papakostas GI, et al. "The relationship between serum folate, vitamin B$_{12}$, and homocysteine levels in major depressive disorder and the timing of improvement with fluoxetine (Prozac)." *International Journal of Neuropsychopharmacology* Dec 2005; 8(4): 523–528 (Epub: 5/9/05).

Papakostas GI, et al. "Serum folate, vitamin B$_{12}$, and homocysteine in major depressive disorder, part 1: predictors of clinical response in fluoxetine-resistant depression." *Journal of Clinical Psychiatry* Aug 2004; 65(8): 1090–1095.

Papakostas GI, et al. "Serum folate, vitamin B$_{12}$, and homocysteine in major depressive disorder, part 2: predictors of relapse during the continuation phase of pharmacotherapy." *Journal of Clinical Psychiatry* Aug 2004; 65(8): 1096–1098.

Pinto J, YP Huang, N Pelliccione, et al. "Cardiac sensitivity to the inhibitory effects of chlorpromazine, imipramine and amitriptyline upon formation of favins." *Biochemical Pharmacology* Nov 1982; 31(21): 3495–3499.

Rush, AJ, MH Trivedi, SR Wisniewski, et al. "Bupropion-SR, sertraline, or venlafaxine-XR after failure of SSRIs for depression." *New England Journal of Medicine* 2006; 354: 1231–1242.

Shamir E, Y Barak, I Shalman, et al. "Melatonin treatment for tardive dyskinesia: a double-blind, placebo-controlled, crossover study." *Archives of General Psychiatry* 2001; 58: 1049–1052.

Stewart JW, et al. "Phenelzine-induced pyridoxine deficiency." *Journal of Clinical Psychopharmacology* Aug 1984; 4(4): 225–226.

Stoll AL, GS Sachs, BM Cohen, et al, "Choline in the treatment of rapid-cycling bipolar disorder: clinical and neurochemical findings in lithium-treated patients." *Biological Psychiatry* Dec 1996; 40(5): 382–390.

Taylor MJ, SM Carney, GM Goodwin, et al. "Folate for depressive disorders: systematic review and meta-analysis of randomized controlled trials." *Journal of Psychopharmacology* Jun 2004; 18(2): 251–256.

Tiemeier H, HR van Tuijl, A Hofman, et al. "Vitamin B$_{12}$, folate, and homocysteine in depression: the Rotterdam study." *American Journal of Psychiatry* Dec 2002; 159: 2099–2101.

Vieth R, et al. "Randomized comparison of the effects of the vitamin D$_3$ adequate intake versus 100 mcg (4000 IU) per day on biochemical responses and the wellbeing of patients." *Nutrition Journal* July 2004; 3: 8.

Chapter 8

Baum CL, J Selhub, and IH Rosenberg. "Antifolate actions of sulfasalazine on intact lymphocytes." *Journal of Laboratory and Clinical Medicine* 1981; 97: 779–784.

Baum MK, JJ Javier, E Mantero-Atienza, et al. "Zidovudine-associated adverse reactions in a longitudinal study of asymptomatic HIV-1-infected homosexual males." *Acquired Immune Deficiency Syndrome* 1991; 4(12): 1218–1226.

Blum M, E Kitai, Y Ariel, et al. "Oral contraceptive lowers serum magnesium." *Harefuah* 1991; 121(10): 363–364.

Boshes B. "Sinemet and the treatment of Parkinsonism." *Annals of Internal Medicine* Mar 1981; 94(3): 364–370.

Bourgeois BF, WE Dodson, and JA Ferrendelli. "Interactions between primidone, carbamazepine, and nicotinamide." *Neurology* Oct 1982; 32(10): 1122–1126.

Conly J and K Stein. "Reduction of vitamin K_2 concentrations in human liver associated with the use of broad-spectrum antimicrobials." *Clinical and Investigative Medicine* 1994; 17(6): 531–539.

Dalakas MC, ME Leon-Monzon, I Bernardini, et al. "Zidovudine-induced mitochondrial myopathy is associated with muscle carnitine deficiency and lipid storage." *Annals of Neurology* 1994; 35(4): 482–487.

Drummond, E. *Overcoming Anxiety without Tranquilizers.* New York: Dutton Books, 1997.

Gorbach SL. "Bengt E. Gustafsson memorial lecture: function of the normal human microflora." *Scand J Infect Dis Suppl* 1986; 49: 17–30.

Famularo G, S Moretti, et al. "Acetyl-carnitine deficiency in AIDS patients with neurotoxicity on treatment with antiretroviral nucleoside analogues." *AIDS* Feb 1997; 11(2): 185–190.

Granerus AK, R Jagenburg, and A Svanborg. "Kaliuretic effect of L-dopa treatment in Parkinsonian patients. *Acta Med Scand.* 1977; 201(4): 291–297.

Harper JM, AJ Levine, DL Rosenthal, et al. "Erythrocyte folate levels, oral contraceptive use and abnormal cervical cytology." *Acta Cytologica* 1994; 38(3): 324–330.

Hart AM, AD Wilson, C Montovani, et al. "Acetyl-l-carnitine: a pathogenesis-based treatment for HIV-associated antiretroviral toxic neuropathy. *AIDS* 2004; 18(11): 1549–1560.

Haspels AA, HJ Bennink, and WH Schreurs. "Disturbance of tryptophan metabolism and its correction during oestrogen treatment in postmenopausal women," *Maturitas* 1978; 1(1): 15–20.

Ilias I, I Manoli, MR Blackman, et al. "L-carnitine and acetyl-l-carnitine in the treatment of complications associated with HIV infection and antiretroviral therapy." *Mitochondrion* 2004; 4(2–3): 163–168.

Kishi H, T Kishi, and K Folkers. "Bioenergetics in clinical medicine, III, inhibition of coenzyme Q_{10}-enzymes by clinically used antihypertensive drugs." *Research Communications in Chemical Pathology and Pharmacology* 1975; 12(3): 533–540.

Kowalczyk L. "FDA requests anticonvulsants be reexamined." *The Boston Globe,* April 20, 2005.

Lader, M. "Benzodiazepines—the opiate of the masses?" *Neuroscience* 1978; 3: 159–165.

Lader, M. "Dependence on benzodiazepines." *Journal of Clinical Psychiatry* 1983; 44: 121–127.

Leeb BF, G Witzmann, E Ogris, et al. "Folic acid and cyanocobalamin levels in serum and erythrocytes during low-dose methotrexate therapy of rheumatoid arthritis and psoriatic arthritis patients." *Clinical and Experimental Rheumatology* 1995; 13(4): 459–463.

Meyrick T, R Payne, MM Black, et al. "Isoniazid-induced pellagra." *British Medical Journal* 1981; 283: 287–288.

Muller T, T Buttner, AF Gholipour, and W Kuhn. "Coenzyme Q_{10} supplementation provides mild symptomatic benefit in patients with Parkinson's disease." *Neuroscience Lett.* 2003; 341(3): 201–204.

Oster, G, et al. "Benzodiazepines and the risk of traffic accidents." *American Journal of Public Health* 1990; 80: 1467–1470.

Paltiel O, J Falutz, M Veilleux, et al. "Clinical correlates of subnormal vitamin B_{12} levels in patients infected with the human immunodeficiency virus." *American Journal of Hematology* 1995; 49(4): 318–322.

Pelton R, JB Lavalle, and EB Hawkins. *Drug-Induced Nutrient Depletion Handbook 1999–2000.* Hudson, OH: Lexi-Comp, Inc, 1999.

Race TF, IC Paes, and WW Faloon. "Intestinal malabsorption induced by oral colcichine." *American Journal of Medical Sciences* 1970; 259(1): 32–41.

Sanders ME. "Considerations for use of probiotic bacteria to modulate human health." *American Journal of Nutrition* 2000;130: 384S–390S.

Schneider RE and L Beeley. "Megaloblastic anaemia associated with sulphasalazine treatment." *British Medical Journal* 1977; 1: 1683.

Seelig MS. "Interrelationship of magnesium and estrogen in cardiovascular and bone disorders, eclampsia, migraine, and premenstrual syndrome." *Journal of the American College of Nutrition* 1993; 12(4): 442–458.

Sima AA, M Calvani, M Mehra, et al. "Acetyl-l-carnitine improves pain, nerve regeneration, and vibratory perception in patients with chronic diabetic neuropathy: an analysis of two randomized, placebo-controlled trials." *Diabetes Care* 2005; 28(1): 89–94.

Stevens CE and ID Hume. "Contributions of microbes in vertebrate gastrointestinal tract to production and conservation of nutrients." *Physiological Review* 1998; 78(2): 494–427.

Surtees RR and K Hyland. "L-3,4-dihydroxyphenylalanine (levodopa) lowers central nervous system S-adenosylmethionine concentrations in humans." *Journal of Neurology, Neurosurgery & Psychiatry* Jul 1990; 53(7): 569–572.

Tinetti, ME, et al. "Risk factors for falls among elderly persons living in the community." *New England Journal of Medicine* 1988; 319: 1701–1707.

Wasser S. "Medicinal mushrooms as a source of anti-tumor and immunomodulating polysaccharides." *Applied Microbiology and Biotechnology* Nov 2002; 60(3): 258–258.

Webb JL. "Nutritional effects of oral contraceptive use: a review." *Journal of Reproductive Medicine* 1980; 25(4): 150–156.

Index

oil, 24
Fluctin, 118
Fluoxetine, 118
Fluphenazine, 137
Flurazepam, 139
Fluvastatin, 65
Folate. *See* Folic acid.
Folex PFS, 147
Folic acid, 32, 45, 49–50, 52, 56, 64, 74,
    78, 85–86, 93, 100, 105, 110, 115,
    121, 124, 128, 139, 144, 146, 148,
    149, 152
Food, 19–21, 21–28, 95–111, 114–116
    antioxidant-rich, 26–27
    color of, 27
    depression and, 114–116
    fried, 25
    low-glycemic, 43
    raw, 109
    See also Diet.
Food allergies, 83
    rheumatoid arthritis and, 83
Fontex, 118
Fosamax, 2, 150
Fox, Michael J., 147
Foxglove, 7
Free radicals, 25–26, 72
Fruits, 26–27, 35, 141
Functional medicine, 156
Furosemide, 74

Gabapentin, 135
Gamma-aminobutyric acid (GABA),
    114, 115, 139, 140
Gamma-linolenic acid. *See* GLA.
Garlic, 79
Gastroesophageal reflux disease. *See*
    GERD.
Gastrointestinal tract. *See* GI tract.
Gavison, 100
Gelusil, 100
Gemfibrozil, 64
Genetics, 16
Geodon, 137
GERD, 97–99
    case studies, 97–98
GI tract, 14–16, 95–99
    case studies, 95

bleeding, 81–82, 85
Ginger, 90, 94
Gittleman, Ann Louise, 29
GLA, 24
Gladem, 118
Glenmullen, Joseph, 120
Glimepiride, 45, 46
Glipizide, 45
Glucophage, 44
Glucophage XR, 44
Glucotrol, 45
Glucosamine/Chondroitin, 89, 94
Glucose. *See* Blood sugar.
Glucovance, 44
Glutamine, 115, 141
Glyburide, 45
Glycemic index, 22, 46
Glycemic load, 22
Glynase, 45
Glyset, 46
Gout, 143
Grapeseed, extract, 79
Graveline, Duane "Doc," 67
Guanfacine, 76
Guided imagery, 127

H2 blockers, 100–101, 106–108
H. pylori, 99, 102
Halcion, 139
Haldol, 137
Haloperidol, 137
Harpagophytum procumbens. See
    Devil's claw.
Harvard, 120
    Medical School, 10
    School of Public Health 23
Hawkins, David, 138
Hawthorn, 79
Heart disease, 40, 57–79
    drugs for, 63–79
Heart attacks, 59
Heartburn, 95–99, 108–109
    preventing, 108–109
Heber, David, 27
Heidelberg Test, 98
Herbs, 7, 27–28, 142
    standardized, 35
    supplements, 77

About the Author

Hyla Cass, M.D., is an often-quoted expert in the field of integrative medicine and psychiatry. In her clinical practice, writings, lectures, and nationwide media appearances, Dr. Cass combines the best of leading-edge natural medicine with modern science. She is a former Assistant Clinical Professor at UCLA School of Medicine and the author of several groundbreaking books, including *Natural Highs* (Avery, 2003) and *8 Weeks to Vibrant Health* (McGraw-Hill, 2004). Other books include *User's Guide to Ginkgo* (2002), *User's Guide to Vitamin C* (2002) and *User's Guide to Herbal Remedies* (2004)—all published by Basic Health Publications. For more information, see her website, www.drcass.com.